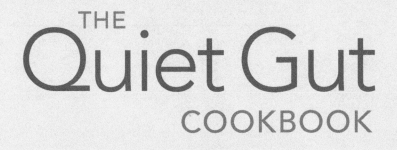

THE Quiet Gut
COOKBOOK

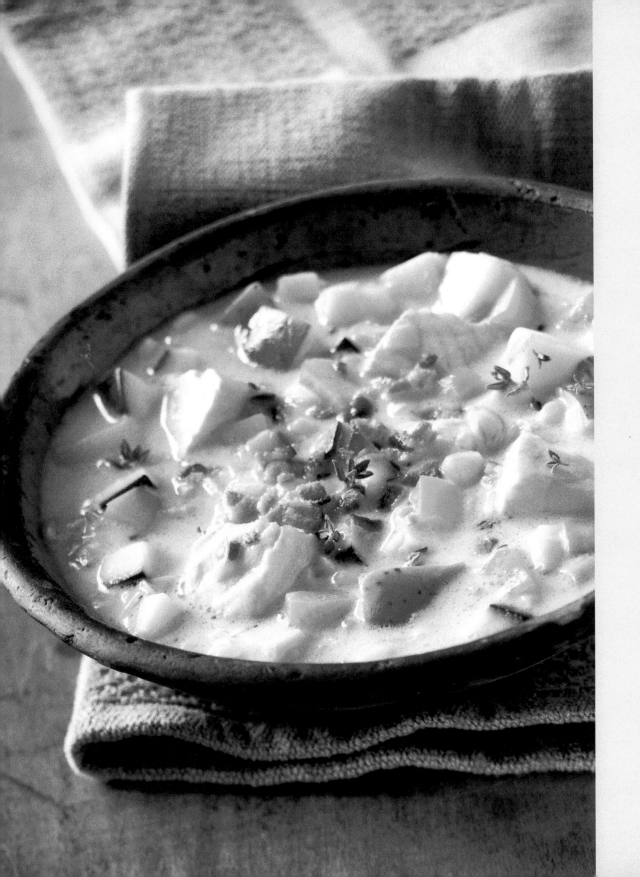

THE
Quiet Gut
COOKBOOK

135 Easy Low-FODMAP Recipes
to Soothe Symptoms of
IBS, IBD, and Celiac Disease

SONOMA
PRESS

Front cover photos: Dorling Kindersley/Getty Images. Back cover, clockwise from top left: Tanya Zouev/Stockfood; Leigh Beisch/Stockfood; Clive Streeter/Stockfood.

Interior photos: Alan Richardson/Stockfood, p. 2; Valerie Janssen/Stockfood, p. 6 (top right); Lumina/Stocksy, p. 6 (bottom left); La Food–Thomas Dhellemmes/Stockfood, p. 11 (left); Borislav Zhuykov/Stocksy, p. 11 (right); Linda; Pugliese/Stockfood, p. 12; John Hay/Stockfood, p. 24; Canan Czemmel/Stocksy, p. 31 (left); Eising Studio–Food Photo & Video/Stockfood, p. 36; mee productions/Stocksy, p. 42; Amélie Roche/Stockfood, p. 51; Canan Czemmel/Stocksy, p. 56; Tanya Zouev/Stockfood, p. 63; Jonathan Gregson/Stockfood, p. 68; Julia Cawley/Stockfood, p. 75; Michael St. John/Stockfood, p. 82; Mikkel Adsbo/Stockfood, p. 89; Tanya Zouev/Stockfood, p. 94; Clive Streeter/Stockfood, p. 101; Mark Thomas/Stockfood, p. 104; Rua Castilho/Stockfood, p. 109; Carmen Mariani/Stockfood, p. 112; Eising Studio–Food Photo & Video/Stockfood, p. 119; Leigh Beisch/Stockfood, p. 124; Alan Richardson/Stockfood, p. 134; Michael Wissing/Stockfood, p. 143; Uwe Bender/Stockfood, p. 152; Tim Winter; Stockfood, p. 160; Rafael Pranschke/Stockfood, p. 169; Keller & Keller Photography/Stockfood, p. 176; Louise Lister/Stockfood, p. 184; Rua Castilho/Stockfood, p. 193; Petr Gross/Stockfood, p. 200; Valérie Lhomme/Stockfood, p. 207; Tower Above Studio/Stockfood, p. 212; Klaus Arras/Stockfood, p. 220; Illanique van Aswegen/Stockfood, p. 225; Bruce James/Stockfood, p. 230; Westend61/Stockfood, p. 237; Jean-Christophe Riou/Stockfood, p. 244. All other photos Shutterstock.com.

ISBN: Print 978-1-942411-01-7 | eBook 978-1-942411-02-4

Contents

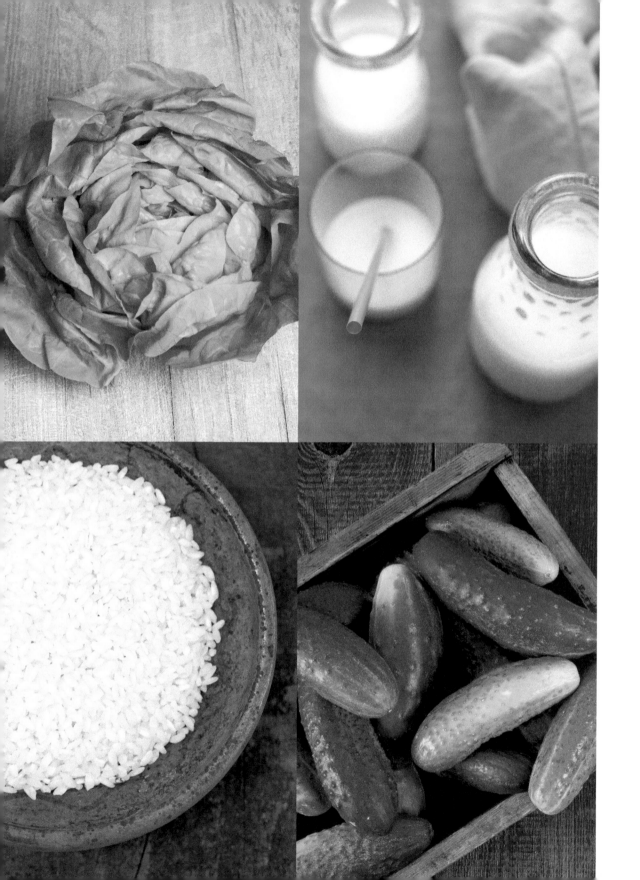

Introduction

If you suffer from a chronic digestive condition, you are likely all too familiar with the uncomfortable and sometimes embarrassing symptoms associated with an inflamed gut. Gas, bloating, abdominal distention, discomfort, pain, diarrhea, and constipation are the hallmarks of irritable bowel syndrome (IBS), inflammatory bowel disease (IBD), celiac disease, and other functional gastrointestinal disorders (FGID). For some sufferers, these symptoms are so extreme they can lead to social isolation, depression, and emotional anguish. It may be a relief, then, to know that a dietary solution is available, one that offers you the chance to control your symptoms without relying exclusively on expensive medication or a bewildering array of supplements.

You may already suspect that certain foods exacerbate your symptoms and have even tried various elimination diets to pinpoint your sensitivities. Cutting out foods like red meat, dairy, or gluten may have provided some relief, but you may not be certain of all the foods that trigger your symptoms. Ongoing research since the late 1990s suggests the culprit may be certain short-chain carbohydrates, commonly referred to as FODMAPs. Unfortunately for those who cannot easily digest these carbohydrates, FODMAPs are found in many everyday foods. The good news is that there are delicious and satisfying meals you can make that won't plunge your body into digestive distress. *The Quiet Gut Cookbook* is filled with low-FODMAP recipes to help you soothe your gut and ease your symptoms. This book also offers a basic elimination diet to help you identify which foods are particularly troubling for your digestive system, thereby allowing you to modify your personal diet so that you can eat in a way that is satisfying and helpful. Although the low-FODMAP diet is not designed for long-term use, it provides you with invaluable information about your digestive system. By uncovering your personal food triggers, you gain the knowledge you need to modify your diet in a way that is practical and sustainable. The low-FODMAP diet may not cure IBS or IBD, but it can help you control your symptoms so that your condition is less disruptive to your overall well-being.

So what exactly are FODMAPs? *FODMAP* is an acronym that stands for *fermentable oligosaccharides, disaccharides, monosaccharides,* and *polyols.* These are carbohydrates that absorb water in the small intestine and pass through to the large intestine where they rapidly ferment as naturally occurring gut bacteria consume them. This fermentation process releases gas. It is the combination of excess water and gas that can create abdominal pain or discomfort, flatulence, bloating or abdominal distention, inconsistent or excessive bowel movements, diarrhea, or constipation.

Australian dietitian Sue Shepherd was the first to examine the FODMAP connection to digestive distress. During the course of her search for methods to relieve the gastrointestinal symptoms of celiac disease, she began experimenting with a diet that strictly limited or eliminated FODMAPs and discovered that it could provide marked improvement to the health and quality of life of celiac patients, since an estimated 40 percent of celiac sufferers experience IBS symptoms. The diet proved so helpful that Shepherd joined forces with Professor Peter Gibson at Melbourne's Monash University to conduct further studies. Together, they found that a low-FODMAP diet significantly reduced digestive symptoms—including bloating, gas, pain and discomfort, diarrhea, and constipation—for 75 percent of subjects with IBS. Since then, Shepherd and Gibson have begun to study the effects of FODMAPs on sufferers of IBD and other gastrointestinal disorders, who often have symptoms that overlap with those of IBS. The researchers found that when sufferers of digestive disorders eliminate FODMAPs from their diet, many can greatly decrease or even eliminate certain symptoms altogether. One study from the Monash researchers showed positive symptom management for people with IBD, a promising start to what is admittedly still very early research.

Removing FODMAPs from your diet may sound like a relatively simple solution, but these potentially troublesome carbohydrates are found in many everyday foods like apples, cherries, beets, cauliflower, leeks, onions, garlic, mushrooms, wheat, soy, barley, beans, milk, cashews, and honey, just to name a few. Following a low-FODMAP diet requires determination, research, and a lot of forethought. On the plus side, this diet does not require more than a couple of months to follow, and the knowledge you gain from your elimination diet may benefit you for a lifetime.

Right now you might be feeling overwhelmed at the thought of making a major dietary and lifestyle change. Fortunately, there is help and hope available. This book provides you with information and advice to help you make this transition as easily as possible. You'll discover more than 135 delicious low-FODMAP recipes created to help you reduce or eliminate symptoms. The recipes eschew all of the high-FODMAP foods and include only limited amounts of moderate-FODMAP foods. Nearly all the recipes are gluten free and most are free of other common food allergens, including soy, eggs, dairy, nuts, and shellfish. Those recipes that do use these ingredients offer substitution tips for adapting the recipe to suit your dietary needs.

In addition to offering a wealth of delicious, easy-to-prepare, family-friendly recipes that are low in FODMAPs to ease the shared symptoms of IBS, IBD, and celiac disease, this book presents a host of tools that will ease your transition to a low-FODMAP diet, including:

- Detailed charts of foods that are low, moderate, or high in FODMAPs, including recommended serving-size limitations for moderate-FODMAP foods

- A chapter devoted to recipes especially designed to offer post-flare-up relief

- Basic elimination diet guidelines and an elimination-diet meal plan

- A food reintroduction plan to help you gradually bring eliminated foods back into your diet

- A Symptom Tracker to help you document how certain foods affect your symptoms, as well as how to customize your diet and keep tabs on symptom improvement as you adopt the low-FODMAP diet
- A Food Challenges list to help you develop and maintain awareness of your own trigger foods

The Quiet Gut Cookbook can help you reduce and possibly eliminate the symptoms of your chronic digestive conditions as you enjoy appetizing, simple-to-prepare, family-friendly meals. Get ready to embrace a low-FODMAP diet and get back on the track to living your life again.

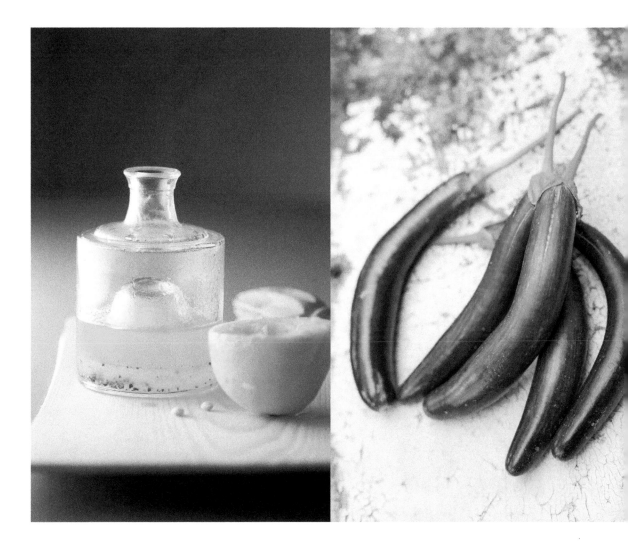

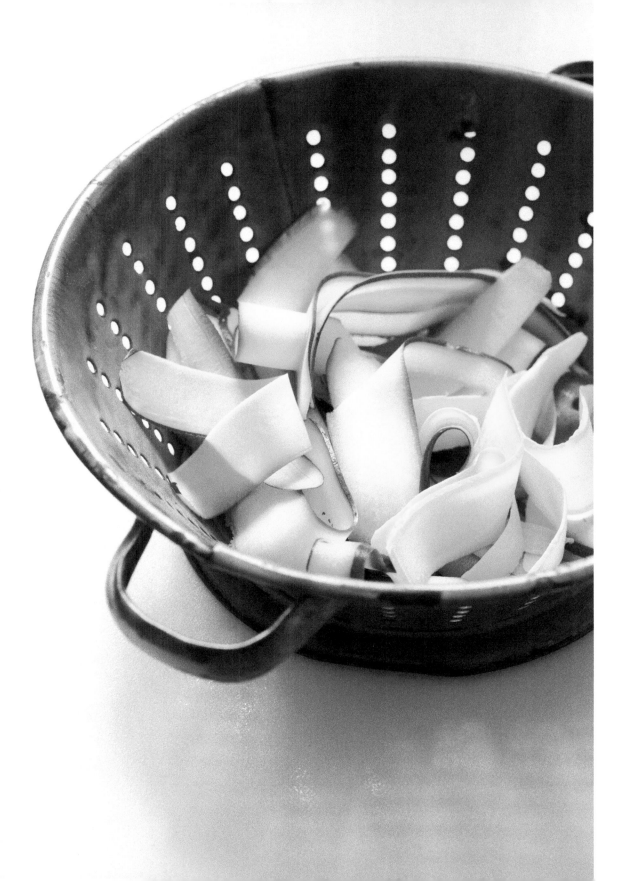

1

Eat to Calm
and Soothe the Gut

A low-FODMAP diet has been used successfully to manage the symptoms of IBS, which are often also present in people with other digestive disorders such as IBD and celiac disease, and it can be invaluable in identifying the personal triggers that cause painful flare-ups. The diet has not been studied for its long-term effects, however, so it is not recommended as a lifelong diet. Plus, it is not always the right diet for everyone with IBS, IBD, or celiac disease. Each of these disorders has a unique profile and specific dietary considerations, and your own health profile may affect the low-FODMAP diet's effect on your symptoms. If you have not yet done so, be sure to consult your primary health care provider if you are experiencing the following symptoms of chronic digestive distress and before making changes to your diet.

Irritable Bowel Syndrome

Irritable bowel syndrome (IBS) is a common disorder shared by 25 to 45 million Americans. The condition affects the large intestine, causing cramping, abdominal pain, bloating, gas, diarrhea, and constipation. According to the Mayo Clinic, a variety of factors can cause IBS, including poor bowel motility (the muscles of the bowel don't contract normally), hypersensitivity (increased sensitivity of the nerves in the bowel), or hormonal or neurotransmitter imbalances affecting the nervous system. While exactly what brings about IBS is not yet fully understood, it is known that triggers—which can include certain foods, stress, or medications—can cause symptoms to appear or worsen.

Celiac Disease

Celiac disease is an inflammatory autoimmune disorder. With this disease, gluten must be completely avoided. Eating gluten (a protein found in wheat, barley, and rye) causes the body's immune system to attack the small intestine. Repeated episodes of this attack damage the lining of the small intestine, eventually compromising its ability to absorb nutrients. According to the National Institute of Diabetes and Digestive and Kidney Diseases, untreated celiac disease can lead to a host of serious health issues including infertility, osteoporosis, anemia, intestinal cancer, and neurological conditions such as epilepsy. The treatment for celiac disease is strict adherence to a completely gluten-free diet.

As with IBD, many people with celiac disease have symptoms that overlap with those of IBS, and a low-FODMAP diet can be helpful in reducing or eliminating those symptoms. A low-FODMAP diet is not completely gluten free, but substitutions can be made to meet the necessary dietary restrictions. If you have celiac disease, be extremely careful about hidden sources of gluten, such as in traditional soy sauce, malt syrup, and popular brands of bouillon cubes. You must also be careful of cross-contamination. Even a few small crumbs on a cutting board or knife can introduce enough gluten into the digestive system to stimulate a reaction.

Inflammatory Bowel Disease

The Mayo Clinic includes a few disorders in its definition of inflammatory bowel disease (IBD). Two of them—ulcerative colitis and Crohn's disease—cause chronic inflammation of the digestive tract and so are addressed in this book. Ulcerative colitis affects the colon (large intestine) and rectum and causes inflammation and ulcers. Crohn's disease most commonly affects the large intestine and the small intestine, but it can produce inflammation of the lining of any part of the digestive tract. The symptoms of IBD typically include severe diarrhea, pain, fatigue, and weight loss. The cause of IBD is still unknown, but treatments include anti-inflammatory medications, immune-system suppressants, antibiotics, and pain relievers.

According to the Crohn's and Colitis Foundation of America, food allergies and food sensitivities do not cause IBD, nor will special diets reverse the effects of these diseases. However, limiting or eliminating poorly digestible carbohydrates may significantly lessen IBS symptoms such as gas, bloating, cramping, and diarrhea, which can help the many IBD patients who also experience IBS symptoms. For these patients, a low-FODMAP diet may be helpful in minimizing discomfort.

It is important to note, though, that a strict low-FODMAP diet may *not* be a good choice for many other people with Crohn's disease or for some people with ulcerative colitis. Both conditions can cause the development of strictures, or a narrowing of the lower small intestine, which can make processing fiber difficult. For these patients, a low-residue or low-fiber diet is important to prevent blockages. Eating FODMAPs may help them maintain fluid in the bowel so that food keeps moving, too.

What Exactly Are FODMAPs?

FODMAPs are certain short-chain carbohydrates that are difficult for the body to absorb. They also ferment easily in the gastrointestinal tract, hence the first letter of the acronym: *Fermentable*. While all FODMAPs are carbohydrates, not all carbohydrates contain FODMAPs. Overall, FODMAPs fall into four categories, which are described in the following sections. Each description contains information about the number of grams per serving that indicates a high-FODMAP food. You will not need to memorize these numbers to make use of this book. Instead, you will find the lists of low-, moderate-, and high-FODMAP foods in Appendix A to be more helpful and perhaps easier to remember.

DIETARY CONSIDERATIONS
FOR IBS, IBD, AND CELIAC DISEASE

Disorder	Description	Dietary Considerations
IBS	A disorder of the large intestine that causes cramping, abdominal pain, bloating, gas, diarrhea, and constipation.	Consider FODMAP elimination and reintroduction diet to identify personal triggers and to manage symptoms. Minimize to your personal tolerance the following foods: caffeine, alcohol, high-fat foods, spicy foods, and foods that can cause gas or bloating, such as beans, broccoli, dried fruits, or bread.
Crohn's disease	A chronic inflammatory disease that most commonly affects the end of the small intestine (the ileum) and the beginning of the colon but can affect any part of the gastrointestinal tract from the mouth to the anus. Symptoms include abdominal pain, cramping, gas, bloating, and diarrhea.	Consider FODMAP elimination and reintroduction diet to identify personal triggers and to manage symptoms that overlap with IBS. Avoid caffeine, alcohol, hard-to-digest foods like seeds and popcorn, high-fat foods, and high-sugar foods. However, if you have strictures in the small intestine, a low-fiber diet that *includes* FODMAPs is recommended.
Ulcerative Colitis	A chronic inflammatory disease of the colon (large intestine). Symptoms include abdominal pain, cramping, gas, bloating, and diarrhea.	Consider FODMAP elimination and reintroduction diet to identify personal triggers and to help manage symptoms that overlap with IBS. Avoid caffeine, alcohol, high-fat foods, fried foods, high-fiber foods, and dried fruits. Note that if you have strictures, a low-fiber diet that *includes* FODMAPs is recommended.
Celiac Disease	An autoimmune disorder in which any amount of gluten in the diet causes damage to the lining of the small intestine. Symptoms include fatigue, bloating, abdominal pain, gas, and diarrhea.	Eat a completely gluten-free diet. Consider FODMAP elimination and reintroduction diet to help manage symptoms that overlap with those of IBS.

Oligosaccharides

Oligosaccharides are a type of FODMAP that includes both fructans and galacto-oligosaccharides (GOS). *Fructans* are indigestible, water-soluble fibers of fructose molecules. They are found in many everyday foods, including wheat, rye, onions, garlic, dried chickpeas, dried lentils, other dried beans, pistachios, cashews, and watermelons. Because fructans exist in so many commonly consumed foods and are malabsorbed by everyone, they can be a common trigger. A cereal or grain is considered a high-FODMAP food if it contains more than 0.3 grams of fructans per serving. For other foods, the amount is more than 0.2 grams per serving.

GOS are galactose molecules joined by fructose and glucose. Like fructans, GOS are indigestible and can cause digestive symptoms, especially for those who already have digestive disorders. They are found in legumes such as black beans, kidney beans, soybeans, chickpeas, and lentils. For legumes, 0.2 grams per serving is considered a high-FODMAP level.

Disaccharides

The disaccharide of concern as a FODMAP is *lactose*. This double sugar (glucose and galactose) is found in animal milk, including cow, sheep, and goat. Fortunately, not all dairy products contain high quantities of lactose. If you have trouble digesting lactose, you will likely want to avoid milk, yogurt, ice cream, and soft cheeses (cottage cheese, ricotta), but you may have little or no problem eating small amounts of whipped cream, hard cheeses, and butter, which contain very low levels of the disaccharide. You may also enjoy lactose-free milk as a more tolerable option, too.

Lactose is broken down in the small intestine by the enzyme lactase. If you are lactose-intolerant, that means your body does not produce sufficient lactase to break down large quantities of lactose. Reducing your intake of lactose while cutting down on other FODMAPs in your diet can help minimize symptoms. Even lactose-intolerant people can often comfortably consume up to 4 grams of lactose per serving of food; any more than this amount might cause unwanted symptoms.

Monosaccharides

Fructose (or fruit sugar) is the FODMAP of greatest concern among the monosaccharides. All fruits contain fructose. The simple sugar is also in cane sugar, honey, high-fructose corn syrup, agave nectar, and some vegetables (sugar snap peas, artichokes, asparagus). Individuals with Crohn's disease typically have a higher incidence of fructose malabsorption than people with IBS, so if you have Crohn's, you may want to pay extra attention to foods that contain excess fructose.

Foods that contain excess fructose are not easily absorbed and can exacerbate digestive symptoms. The presence of glucose, however, helps the body absorb fructose. If the food has .15 grams more fructose than glucose, then it would be deemed a source of excess fructose. However, if a food has an equal amount of fructose and glucose, you should be able to digest it without discomfort. As long as they are limited to one serving per meal, fruits such as kiwifruits, bananas, oranges, tangerines, and grapes can be part of a low-FODMAP diet.

Polyols

Polyols are sugar alcohols. Sugar alcohols exist naturally in some fruits and vegetables such as apples, apricots, blackberries, cauliflower, mushrooms, nectarines, peaches, pears, snow peas, and watermelons. They are also used as artificial sweeteners in processed or "sugar-free" foods, especially in candy and chewing gum. Sorbitol, mannitol, maltitol, xylitol, polydextrose, and isomalt are all polyols.

The whole concept of FODMAPs may seem confusing, and the most important points are as follows:

- Many everyday foods contain FODMAPs.

- The low-FODMAP diet is an elimination diet that is not designed to be followed long term, but rather to be used as a learning diet for identifying a person's unique symptom triggers.

- Many people have trouble absorbing certain FODMAPs (fructans, GOS, and polyols) or experience negative effects when they consume foods that contain them.

- Foods containing fructans, GOS, and polyols are best avoided completely during the initial phase of a low-FODMAP diet.

- Even people who are sensitive to certain FODMAPs may be able to consume some FODMAPs in moderation without experiencing symptoms.

- Certain people are unable to digest lactose or fructose. An elimination diet and reintroduction plan can help you determine if you need to avoid these ingredients long term.

- Some FODMAPs may be more troublesome for you than others. Again, an elimination diet and reintroduction plan can help you pinpoint the FODMAPs to which you are most sensitive and customize an eating plan that will lessen and possibly eliminate your adverse symptoms.

- Sensitivity to FODMAPs can change over time, so periodic reintroduction of FODMAPs is recommended to gauge current tolerance levels.

COMMON SOURCES OF FODMAPS

FODMAP	Examples of Common Sources
Oligosaccharides (fructans)	Onions, garlic, leeks, shallots, wheat, graham flour, pasta, rye, persimmons, watermelon, chicory, dandelion greens, artichokes, beets, asparagus, okra, Brussels sprouts, wheat
Galacto-oligosaccharides (GOS)	Dried lentils and chickpeas (garbanzo beans), hummus, kidney beans, pinto beans, peas, whole soybeans
Disaccharides (lactose)	Cow's milk, sheep's milk, goat's milk, ice cream, yogurt, sour cream, soft cheeses (such as ricotta and cottage cheese)
Monosaccharides (fructose)	High-fructose corn syrup, honey, agave nectar, apples, pears, mangos, asparagus, cherries, watermelons, fruit juice, sugar snap peas
Polyols	Xylitol, mannitol, sorbitol, glycerol, isomalt, lactitol, maltitol, apples, apricots, celery, peaches, nectarines, pears, plums, prunes, cherries, avocados, blackberries, lychees, cauliflower, mushrooms

How Can a Low-FODMAP Diet Help?

A low-FODMAP diet is a learning diet that can be tailored to create your personal lifestyle plan. Far from a diet of deprivation, the eating plan is customizable, allowing you to enjoy your life and your meals more fully by helping you manage your digestive symptoms—whether you have IBS or have IBD or celiac disease with overlapping IBS symptoms. A low-FODMAP diet allows many sufferers of IBS and other digestive disorders to alleviate their gastrointestinal discomfort, and, consequently, the accompanying stress and anxiety caused by experiencing unpredictable symptoms. Perhaps even more important, many people with chronic digestive disorders find that a low-FODMAP diet helps reduce some of their reliance on drugs and other medical treatments.

For best results, begin your low-FODMAP diet with a strict limitation of your intake of FODMAPs. This level of restriction will give you a better sense of whether or not this diet can assist you with symptom control. Your Elimination Diet Meal Plan, on page 27, will guide you through this phase. Once you've removed the high-FODMAP foods from your diet, you are likely to not only enjoy a reduction of negative symptoms but also find that as your body calms or heals over time, your tolerance for many previously off-limits foods will increase.

All of the recipes in this book exclude foods high in FODMAPs and limit the quantity of low- and moderate-FODMAP ingredients. This makes it easy for you to design a meal plan that is low in FODMAPs while also limiting the overall number of low-FODMAP foods you eat. The effects of FODMAPs are cumulative, so eating small quantities of several low-FODMAP foods in a single meal can be just as detrimental as eating a large quantity of a single high-FODMAP food.

Once you've eliminated high-FODMAP foods from your diet and reduced or eliminated your symptoms, you can strategically reintroduce foods into your diet. Use the Symptom Tracker on page 32 and the Food Challenges list on page 34 to help you get a handle on which FODMAP-containing foods affect you negatively and which have minimal or no effect. Over time, you'll develop a personalized eating plan that you can use to manage your symptoms for the rest of your life.

Guidelines for Following a Low-FODMAP Diet

• Be prepared. Before making any major change to your diet, discuss your plans with your doctor for the best results. If you suspect that you might have celiac disease, it is essential that you get the proper medical screening before eliminating gluten from your diet. You might also have other conditions that affect what you should and shouldn't eat, and your doctor can help navigate these issues.

• Study the food lists on pages 245 to 250. Spend some time thinking about which of your favorite foods you may need to eliminate from your diet and what foods you can substitute for them. Get a general sense of what the low-FODMAP diet will look like in practice. This is the perfect time to go through your kitchen cupboards, refrigerator, and freezer to clear out any off-limits foods and make a shopping trip to load up on permissible foods.

• Follow the low-FODMAP diet strictly for four weeks. After this period you might be able to begin reintroducing some foods to your diet, but it's important to reduce your dietary levels of FODMAPs as much as possible to identify which foods are problematic.

• Use the Symptom Tracker on page 32 to document your symptoms over these weeks. If you still experience troublesome symptoms after four weeks of the diet, continue the strict elimination phase for two more weeks. If, after six weeks, you still have significant symptoms, see your doctor to determine another plan of action. If your symptoms have been significantly reduced or eliminated, begin reintroducing foods by following the food reintroduction plan on page 33.

• Remember that the effects of FODMAPs are cumulative. While you might be able to eat small quantities of FODMAPs one at a time, their effects in bulk can gang up on you. In other words, eating small quantities of several different FODMAPs in one meal can be just as detrimental as eating a large quantity of one FODMAP.

- Be aware that many foods considered permissible on the low-FODMAP diet, including virtually all of the permitted fruits and vegetables, contain low levels of FODMAPs. Eating these foods in moderation is generally fine, but it's advisable not to consume more than one serving of each of these foods per meal. An example of one serving is ¾ cup cantaloupe or 1 cup green beans.

Preparation and commitment are the keys to any successful lifestyle change. Since FODMAPs are found in such a wide range of everyday foods, eliminating them or strictly reducing them in your diet will be no small task. The best guideline is to study the list of foods containing high and moderate levels of FODMAPs and identify which of these foods are present in your current diet. A registered dietitian who is knowledgeable about FODMAPs can help make this process easier. Most people will need to do a major diet overhaul to eliminate these high-FODMAP foods and replace them with low- or moderate-FODMAP foods. Once you've achieved this step, you will likely find the major improvement in your symptoms to be motivation enough to keep you going. Eventually the diet will become second nature.

Five Tips for Success

Switching to a low-FODMAP diet takes effort simply because so many common foods contain FODMAPs. Here are a few tips to help ease the process:

- Plan everything. The importance of this tip cannot be overstated. To make your low-FODMAP diet a success, especially during the strict initial phase, you'll need to think ahead regarding every morsel you put in your mouth. That means planning ahead for every meal and snack. If you intend to eat out, check the restaurant's menu in advance to learn what is safe to order. And don't be afraid to ask questions of the waitstaff or to ask for substitutions, if necessary.

- Cook from scratch. Only by cooking for yourself—completely from scratch—can you maintain real control over which ingredients go into the food you eat. You might want to cook some foods in large batches and freeze them in individual servings to be sure you always have suitable meals on hand.

- Be informed. Study the lists of low-, moderate-, and high-FODMAP foods to develop your sense of which foods to gravitate toward and which are off limits. You might want to print out these lists and post them on your refrigerator or some other place where you can easily reference them when you're planning your meals or reaching for a snack.

- Clear out forbidden foods. Eliminating certain foods from your diet will be worlds easier if you take some time at the beginning to eliminate them from your environment. Clean out your kitchen cupboards and refrigerator, as well as your snack drawer at work. Discard any foods on your restricted list so they won't tempt you.

- Stock up. Take the list of low-FODMAP foods with you to the market to help you load up on items permitted on the diet. Be sure to stock your kitchen with the right ingredients for making healthy, delicious low-FODMAP meals. If you're prone to snacking, stock up on low-FODMAP snack foods, as well.

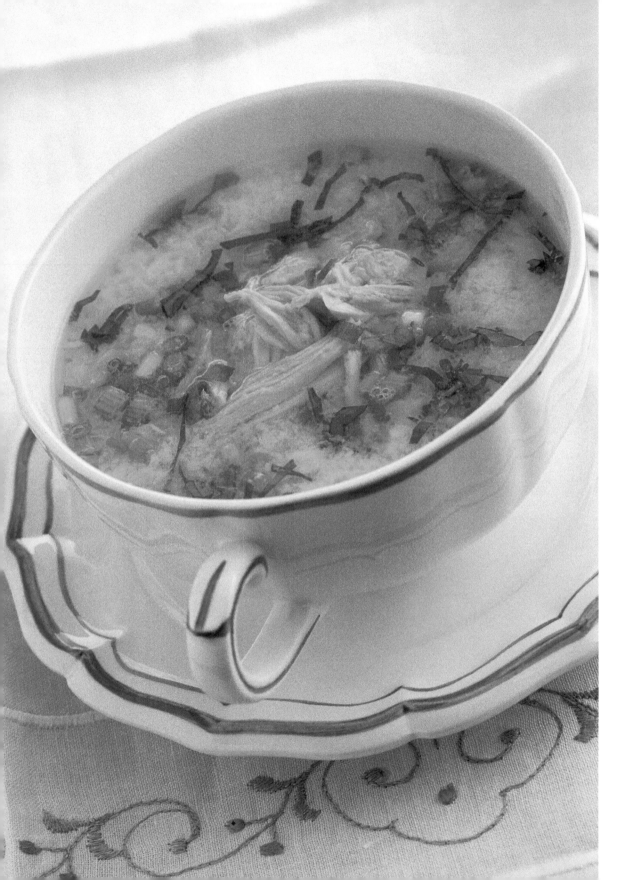

2

Your Basic Elimination Diet and Food Reintroduction Plan

Now that you understand something about what FODMAPs are, which foods contain them, and how they can affect your body, you are ready to begin a basic elimination diet. This guide will help you start off your low-FODMAP diet the right way—by undertaking strict elimination of all high-FODMAP foods. It won't be easy, but rest assured the effort will be worth it. More than likely, you will begin to see a drastic reduction in your digestive symptoms soon after you start making these changes. Once you're past the elimination phase, you can start reintroducing some FODMAP-containing foods to your diet.

The purpose of an elimination diet is to clean all the FODMAPs out of your system. In the course of this process, your body may undergo a period similar to drug withdrawal; for example, you may experience intense cravings for some of the foods you've eliminated, especially wheat, which can be addictive. The good news is that these cravings will begin to subside within three to five days of beginning the low-FODMAP diet.

FODMAP Elimination Diet Guidelines

- For the duration of the elimination diet, eat only low-FODMAP foods. You can find lists of these foods in Appendix A (page 245), and various websites, or download the Monash University Low-FODMAP Diet app, which you can find online (www.med.monash.edu/cecs/gastro/fodmap/iphone-app.html). The latter is updated as new foods are tested for their FODMAP content, making it the most reliable source of current information.

- Read labels carefully. Many processed foods contain unexpected ingredients, so be sure to read the fine print in the ingredient lists, checking for any high-FODMAP foods. A few common high-FODMAP food additives to watch out for include corn syrup, corn sugar, honey, agave nectar, fruit juice, wheat, rye, barley, semolina, fructose, onion and garlic (or spice blends that contain them), artificial flavorings, inulin, sweeteners ending in -ol (maltitol, xylitol, and so on), and legume-based flours (chickpea flour, and so on).

- Avoid processed foods when possible. Because processed foods so often contain problematic ingredients, your best bet is to eat whole foods or foods cooked from scratch.

- Plan ahead for all meals and snacks. By planning all of your meals and snacks in advance, you can avoid accidentally eating high-FODMAP foods. Make a meal plan (or use the one provided on page 27), draw up a comprehensive shopping list, and, ideally, do your shopping for a week at a time.

- Do your research before dining out. Check out the restaurant's menu online beforehand, and if you're unsure of what ingredients a dish contains, don't hesitate to call the restaurant and ask.

- Follow the low-FODMAP meal plan for at least four weeks, while keeping track of your symptoms. If, after four weeks, you are still experiencing symptoms, continue for two additional weeks. If your symptoms persist beyond six weeks on a strict low-FODMAP eating plan, consult with your doctor about other strategies.

By adopting an elimination diet, you can quickly get on top of your symptoms and, in a sense, start with a clean slate. Once you've completed the elimination phase, you can begin to reintroduce certain foods, while carefully monitoring your symptoms, to determine which foods cause severe symptoms and which don't. You may find that just one or two FODMAPs cause the majority of your symptoms while others have little or no negative effect. Ultimately, you'll determine which foods you really need to avoid altogether and which you can eat in moderation.

YOUR ELIMINATION DIET MEAL PLAN

Recipes that are included in this book are indicated with an asterisk (*).

WEEK 1 / *Day One*
Breakfast: Berry and Chia Seed Smoothie*
Lunch: Curried Squash Soup with Coconut Milk*
Dinner: Dijon-Roasted Pork Tenderloin*
Snacks: Spiced Tortilla Chips* with Pico de
  Gallo Salsa*, 2½-inch celery stalk with
  peanut butter

WEEK 1 / *Day Two*
Breakfast: Breakfast Ratatouille with
  Poached Eggs*
Lunch: Kale-Pesto Soba Noodles*
Dinner: Turkey and Sweet Potato Chili*
Snacks: Smoked Trout Brandade* with
  gluten-free crackers, grapes

WEEK 1 / *Day Three*
Breakfast: Crisp rice cereal with ½ sliced banana
  and ½ cup rice milk
Lunch: Mixed green salad with Maple-Mustard
  Vinaigrette,* grilled chicken breast, and
  toasted pecans
Dinner: Quick Shepherd's Pie*
Snacks: Honeydew melon wedges (2) wrapped
  with prosciutto or ham, veggie sticks, and
  Smoky Eggplant Dip*

WEEK 1 / *Day Four*
Breakfast: Oven-Baked Polenta Porridge
  with Strawberries*
Lunch: Chipotle Tofu and Sweet Potato Tacos
  with Guacamole*
Dinner: Vegan Noodles with Gingered
  Coconut Sauce*
Snacks: Maple-Spiced Walnuts,* gluten-free
  toast with peanut butter

Recipes that are included in this book are indicated with an asterisk (*).

WEEK 1 / *Day Five*
Breakfast: Gluten-Free Eggs Benedict*
Lunch: Quinoa-Stuffed Eggplant Roulades
  with Feta and Mint*
Dinner: Chicken Enchiladas*
Snacks: Buttered popcorn, Herbed Veggie-
  and-Tofu Skewers*

WEEK 1 / *Day Six*
Breakfast: Strawberry-Kiwi Smoothie with
  Chia Seeds*
Lunch: Vietnamese Shrimp-and-Herb
  Spring Rolls*
Dinner: Green Chile-Stuffed Turkey Burgers*
Snacks: Lactose-free yogurt, Smoky Eggplant
  Dip* with gluten-free crackers

WEEK 1 / *Day Seven*
Breakfast: Potato Pancakes*
Lunch: Soba noodles with Cilantro-Coconut
  Pesto* and grilled chicken or tofu
Dinner: Pecan-Crusted Maple-Mustard Salmon*
Snacks: Baked Veggie Chips,* hard-boiled eggs

WEEK 2 / *Day One*
Breakfast: Peanut Butter Granola*
Lunch: Lentil-Walnut Burgers*
Dinner: Grilled Halibut Tacos with
  Cabbage Slaw*
Snacks: Grapes, Herbed Polenta "Fries"*
  with Low-FODMAP Spicy Ketchup*

WEEK 2 / *Day Two*
Breakfast: Chia Seed Carrot Cake Pudding*
Lunch: Roast beef and Swiss cheese sandwich
  on gluten-free bread with Homemade
  Mayonnaise,* lettuce, and tomato
Dinner: Arroz con Pollo with Olives, Raisins,
  and Pine Nuts*
Snacks: Olive Tapenade* with gluten-
  free crackers, 2½-inch celery stalk with
  peanut butter

WEEK 2 / *Day Three*
Breakfast: Oven-Baked Zucchini and Carrot
  Fritters with Ginger-Lime Sauce*
Lunch: Turkey and Sweet Potato Chili*
Dinner: Polenta with Roasted Vegetables and
  Spicy Tomato Sauce*
Snacks: Spiced Tortilla Chips* with Pineapple
  Salsa,* carrot sticks

WEEK 2 / *Day Four*
Breakfast: 2 scrambled eggs, 1 slice gluten-free
  toast with butter, ¼ cup sliced strawberries
Lunch: Baked Tofu Báhn Mì Lettuce Wrap*
Dinner: Grilled Carne Asada Tacos with
  Chimichurri Sauce*
Snacks: No-Bake Coconut Cookie Bars,*
  strawberries

WEEK 2 / *Day Five*
Breakfast: Ginger-Berry Rice Milk Smoothie*
Lunch: Lemony Grilled Zucchini with Feta and
  Pine Nuts*
Dinner: Red Snapper with Creole Sauce*
Snacks: Maple-Spiced Walnuts,* Spiced Tortilla
  Chips* with Pico de Gallo Salsa*

Recipes that are included in this book are indicated with an asterisk (*).

WEEK 2 / Day Six
Breakfast: Sausage-Stuffed Kabocha Squash*
Lunch: Watercress Zucchini Soup*
Dinner: Chili-Rubbed Pork Chops with
   Raspberry Sauce*
Snacks: Banana, Smoked Trout Brandade*
   with gluten-free crackers

WEEK 2 / Day Seven
Breakfast: Everything-Free Pancakes*
Lunch: Chicken salad lettuce wraps with
   Homemade Mayonnaise*
Dinner: Risotto with Smoked Salmon and Dill*
Snacks: Chocolate Peanut Butter Cups,*
   strawberries

WEEK 3 / Day One
Breakfast: Orange-Scented Overnight Oatmeal*
Lunch: Spicy Salmon Burgers with
   Cilantro-Lime Mayo*
Dinner: Roasted Chicken, Potatoes, and Kale*
Snacks: Spiced Tortilla Chips* with Pineapple
   Salsa,* carrot sticks

WEEK 3 / Day Two
Breakfast: Breakfast Ratatouille with
   Poached Eggs*
Lunch: Mixed green salad with leftover
   chicken or cooked shrimp with
   Easy Lemon Vinaigrette*
Dinner: Asian-Style Pork Meatballs*
Snacks: Rice cake with peanut butter, cheddar
   cheese with gluten-free crackers

WEEK 3 / Day Three
Breakfast: 2 hard-boiled eggs, ¾ cup honeydew
   melon or cantaloupe
Lunch: Curried Squash Soup with Coconut Milk*
Dinner: Fish and Potato Pie*
Snacks: Popcorn with butter, hard-boiled egg

WEEK 3 / Day Four
Breakfast: Coconut-Banana Oatmeal*
Lunch: Roasted-Veggie Gyros with
   Tzatziki Sauce*
Dinner: Grilled Chicken with
   Maple-Mustard Glaze*
Snacks: Spiced Tortilla Chips* with Spiced
   Carrot Dip,* grapes

WEEK 3 / Day Five
Breakfast: Peanut Butter Granola*
Lunch: Moroccan-Spiced Lentil and
   Quinoa Stew*
Dinner: Ginger-Sesame Grilled Flank Steak*
Snacks: Maple-Spiced Walnuts*

WEEK 3 / Day Six
Breakfast: 2-egg omelet with ham and 1 ounce
   cheddar cheese, ½ cup grapes
Lunch: Lentil-Walnut Burgers*
Dinner: Ginger-Orange Braised Short Ribs*
Snacks: Olive Tapenade* with gluten-free
   crackers, honeydew melon with prosciutto
   or ham

Recipes that are included in this book are indicated with an asterisk (*).

WEEK 3 / *Day Seven*
Breakfast: Quinoa Breakfast Bowl with Basil "Hollandaise" Sauce*

Lunch: Tuna salad with Homemade Mayonnaise* on gluten-free bread with lettuce and tomatoes

Dinner: Italian-Herbed Chicken Meatballs in Broth*

Snacks: Baked Veggie Chips,* steamed veggies with Egg-Free Caesar Dressing*

WEEK 4 / *Day One*
Breakfast: Banana-Rice Milk Smoothie*

Lunch: Romaine lettuce salad with grilled chicken and Egg-Free Caesar Dressing*

Dinner: Thai Sweet Chili Broiled Salmon*

Snacks: Lamb Meatballs,* veggie sticks with Chimichurri Sauce*

WEEK 4 / *Day Two*
Breakfast: Everything-Free Pancakes*

Lunch: Kale-Pesto Soba Noodles*

Dinner: Tempeh Enchiladas with Red Chili Sauce*

Snacks: Strawberries with Whipped Coconut Cream,* cheese and gluten-free crackers

WEEK 4 / *Day Three*
Breakfast: Gluten-Free Eggs Benedict*

Lunch: Chipotle Tofu and Sweet Potato Tacos with Guacamole*

Dinner: Risotto with Smoked Salmon and Dill*

Snacks: Spiced Tortilla Chips* with Smoky Eggplant Dip,* hard-boiled egg

WEEK 4 / *Day Four*
Breakfast: Orange-Scented Overnight Oatmeal*

Lunch: Smoky Corn Chowder with Red Peppers*

Dinner: Spicy Pulled Pork* with Classic Coleslaw*

Snacks: Raspberry-Chia Seed Ice Pops,* popcorn with butter

WEEK 4 / *Day Five*
Breakfast: Huevos Rancheros*

Lunch: Lemony Grilled Zucchini with Feta and Pine Nuts*

Dinner: Steamed Mussels with Saffron-Infused Cream*

Snacks: Herbed Rice Fritters with Parmesan Cheese,* strawberries

WEEK 4 / *Day Six*
Breakfast: Gluten-free cereal, ½ sliced banana, ½ cup rice milk

Lunch: Soba noodles with Cilantro-Coconut Pesto* and grilled chicken or tofu

Dinner: Moroccan-Spiced Lentil and Quinoa Stew*

Snacks: Rice cake with peanut butter, veggie sticks

WEEK 4 / *Day Seven*
Breakfast: Chia Seed Carrot Cake Pudding*

Lunch: Mixed green salad with canned tuna or cooked shrimp with Easy Lemon Vinaigrette*

Dinner: Indian-Spiced Prawns with Coconut Milk*

Snacks: Gluten-Free Lemon-Filled Cookies,* Smoky Eggplant Dip* with carrot sticks

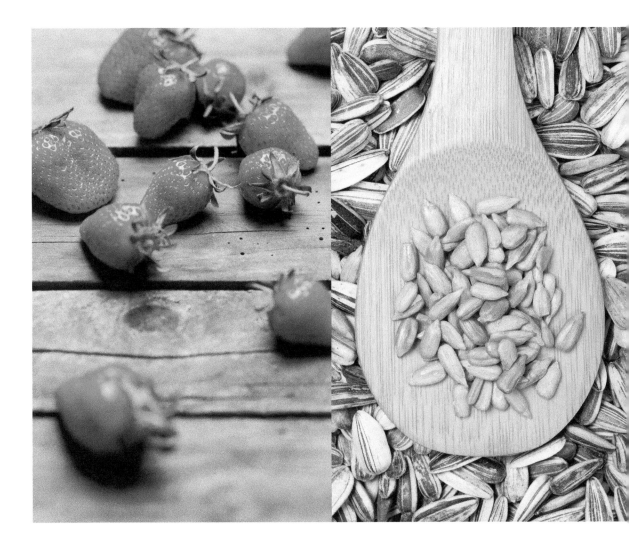

SYMPTOM TRACKER

The key to determining which foods trigger your symptoms is to completely eliminate all potential trigger foods from your diet for a set period of time before carefully reintroducing them one at a time. By keeping track of everything you eat and recording any symptoms in your Symptom Tracker, you'll be able to pinpoint which foods generate unpleasant symptoms and which don't.

Begin by recording your pre-elimination diet symptoms to establish a baseline. Include any symptoms that seem relevant (gas, bloating, abdominal pain, diarrhea, constipation, and any other potentially related symptoms) along with a numerical rating, from 1 to 10, of their severity.

Follow the low-FODMAP diet for a minimum of four weeks. If you continue to experience symptoms after this period, continue for an additional two weeks. At the end of each week, record your symptoms and rate their severity from 1 to 10.

Time Period	Symptoms	Severity
Baseline		
End of Week 1		
End of Week 2		
End of Week 3		
End of Week 4		
End of Week 5		
End of Week 6		

Guidelines for Reintroducing FODMAP-Containing Foods

If, after four to six weeks on the Elimination Diet, your symptoms have improved significantly, start to reintroduce FODMAP-containing foods back into your diet. Reintroduce each of these foods individually as you continue to track your symptoms to determine which foods, if any, trigger your symptoms. Remember to keep the following in mind:

- In order to identify which foods are problematic for you, it is important to reintroduce foods one at a time.

- Because some foods contain multiple FODMAPs, begin by reintroducing foods that contain only one of the five FODMAPs (oligosaccharides, galacto-oligosaccharides, disaccharides, monosaccharides, or polyols). This way you'll be able to pinpoint not just specific foods that trigger your symptoms, but also the specific FODMAPs that do so. Here's a short list of foods that contain only one FODMAP:

    oligosaccharides (fructans): grapefruit, persimmons, wheat bread
    GOS: kidney beans, peas
    disaccharides (lactose): cow's milk, yogurt
    monosaccharides (fructose): fresh figs, mangos, honey
    polyols (sorbitol): blackberries, nectarines
    polyols (mannitol): cauliflower, button mushrooms

- To begin, sample a small quantity of the single-FODMAP-containing food. For instance, try eating ½ cup of pasta made from wheat (which contains oligosaccharides, or fructans) and then track your symptoms over the next 24 hours. If you experience an increase in symptoms, it is likely that fructans are a trigger for you, and you'll need to avoid or severely restrict fructan-containing foods in your diet. Once the symptoms have subsided, you might want to test a smaller quantity of that food to see if you can eat it in limited quantities without negative consequences.

- If you don't experience symptoms, attempt to eat a larger quantity of that food (or another food containing the same type of FODMAP). For instance, you might experiment with 1 cup of pasta or a sandwich made on 2 slices of wheat bread. Again, track your symptoms over the next 24 hours. If you still don't experience negative symptoms, try an even larger quantity of the food. Once you are satisfied that this food is not one of your triggers, move on to the next food or FODMAP type.

• The reintroduction process is slow and may take up to two months to complete. Once you have determined which foods and FODMAP types are your personal triggers, you'll be able to customize your diet in a way that keeps your symptoms under control.

FOOD CHALLENGES

The following chart will serve as a guide to the reintroduction process. It should help you determine which foods to test, while allowing you to keep track of which foods are your triggers and which are safe.

FODMAP Type	Suggested Challenge Foods	Safe Foods	Trigger Foods
Monosaccharides	Honey, agave nectar, mangos, asparagus, sugar snap peas		
Disaccharides	Skim cow's milk, ice cream, low-fat yogurt, ricotta cheese		
Oligosaccharides (fructans)	Onions, garlic, leeks, shallots, wheat couscous, wheat pasta, wheat bread, artichokes, beets		
Galacto-oligosaccharides (GOS)	Kidney beans, peas, soy milk		
Polyols (sorbitol)	Blackberries, nectarines		
Polyols (mannitol)	Cauliflower, button mushrooms		

FOOD CHALLENGE SYMPTOM TRACKER

Use the following chart to track your responses to individual foods as you reintroduce them to your diet.

FODMAP Type	Food/ Serving Size	Date/ Time Eaten	Symptoms	Conclusion

The elimination diet and reintroduction program are hard work, but well worth it. Once you've determined a set of trigger foods, you can customize a diet that will help you keep your symptoms under control. If, after several months, your symptoms are well in hand, you can repeat the food challenges with your trigger foods. After several months of healing time, you may very well find that you are able to tolerate some—or maybe all—of those trigger foods better than you had before. You may find you'll be able to enjoy them in small quantities, or they may no longer trigger your symptoms at all.

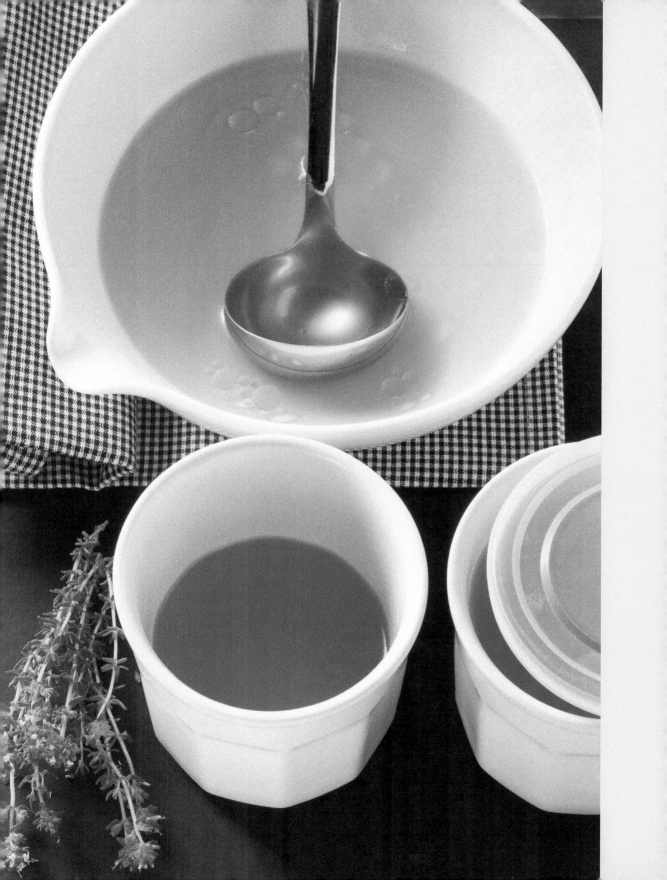

3

Calming Recipes for Flare-Up Relief

Roasted-Vegetable Broth

MAKES ABOUT 2 QUARTS

PREP TIME: 10 MINUTES

COOK TIME: 2 HOURS

Substitution Tip: Feel free to substitute parsnips for some or all of the carrots listed in the recipe, or if you like, simply use them in addition.

PER SERVING

(1 CUP)

Calories: 42
Protein: 1g
Total Fat: 2g
Saturated Fat: 0g
Carbohydrates: 6g
Fiber: 1g
Sodium: 899mg

Nearly every available brand of store-bought vegetable broth contains high-FODMAP onions and garlic, and many are also filled with unnecessary additives. Rich, delicious, highly nutritious, and low-FODMAP homemade vegetable broth is easy to make from scratch. In this version, the vegetables are roasted first to give the broth a deep, intense flavor. The oil is infused with flavor from the onions and garlic, but because the solids are strained and discarded, you don't have to worry about their FODMAP content.

2 tablespoons neutral-flavored oil
1 large onion, sliced
4 cloves garlic, halved
4 large carrots, peeled and quartered
2 tablespoons Garlic Oil (page 202)
1 tablespoon salt (optional)
2 sprigs fresh thyme
1 sprig fresh rosemary
1 bay leaf
6 whole black peppercorns
4 quarts water

1. Preheat the oven to 400°F.

2. In a large skillet, heat the oil over medium-high heat. Add the onions and garlic and cook, stirring, until the onions are softened, about 5 minutes. Using a fine-meshed strainer set over a bowl, strain out the onion and garlic pieces. Discard the solids.

3. On a large, rimmed baking sheet, toss the carrots with the oil. Sprinkle with salt, if using, and spread them out in an even layer. Roast in the preheated oven, stirring occasionally, for 45 to 55 minutes, until the carrots are tender and golden brown.

4. Transfer the roasted carrots to a large stockpot and add the thyme, rosemary, bay leaf, peppercorns, and water. Bring to a boil over high heat. Reduce the heat to low and simmer, uncovered, stirring occasionally, for about 60 minutes. Remove from the heat and let cool.

5. Strain the broth through a fine-meshed strainer, discarding the solids, into glass jars. Cool to room temperature, seal, and refrigerate for up to a week or freeze for up to 3 months.

Chicken-Bone Broth

Substitution Tip: If you can't find chicken feet or simply don't want to use them, substitute 1 additional pound of chicken bones.

PER SERVING

(1 CUP)

Calories: 47
Protein: 7g
Total Fat: 1g
Saturated Fat: 0g
Carbohydrates: 1g
Fiber: 0g
Sodium: 622mg

Your grandmother was onto something with her chicken soup cure-all. Broth made from bones is full of the amino acids arginine, glutamine, glycine, and proline, which soothe the lining of the digestive tract, stimulate the production of healthy stomach acid, and produce an anti-inflammatory effect. Containing gelatin, collagen, and a host of highly absorbable minerals like calcium, magnesium, potassium, and phosphorus, this broth can boost your health. Chicken feet are loaded with even more gelatin, giving your broth a hearty thickness. Many butchers and supermarket chains that process whole chickens have chicken feet, even if they don't display them in the case. You can also purchase frozen chicken feet online. Use the best-quality chicken you can find without added antibiotics; often natural food markets have in-house butchers, too.

1 to 2 pounds chicken bones (2 to 3 chicken carcasses or an equal weight of assorted bones)
½ pound chicken feet
2 medium carrots, cut into 3-inch pieces
2 stalks celery, cut into 3-inch pieces
2 tablespoons white-wine vinegar
1 tablespoon salt (optional)

1. Place all of the ingredients in a 6-quart stockpot or slow cooker. Fill the pot or slow cooker with water. If using a stockpot, bring the liquid to a boil over medium-high heat and then reduce the heat to low, cover, and simmer for at least 4 hours and up to 12. If using a slow cooker , cover and cook on low for at least 10 hours and up to 18 hours. Remove from the heat and allow to cool.

2. Strain the broth through a fine-meshed strainer into glass jars. Let cool to room temperature, cover, and refrigerate for up to a week or freeze for up to 3 months.

Beef-Bone Broth

MAKES 3 TO 4 QUARTS

PREP TIME: 10 MINUTES

COOK TIME: 8 TO 24 HOURS

Substitution Tip: For a bowlful of the same powerful nutrition with a different flavor, substitute lamb bones for the beef bones.

PER SERVING

(1 CUP)

Calories: 40
Protein: 2g
Total Fat: 0g
Saturated Fat: 0g
Carbohydrates: 9g
Fiber: 1g
Sodium: 618mg

Often overlooked and underconsumed in our modern culture, gelatin is a nutritional powerhouse. A great source of protein, it's loaded with collagen and essential amino acids that stimulate the production of healthy stomach acid and have an anti-inflammatory effect. There is no better way to get more gelatin in your diet than slow-cooking beef bones into a rich, flavorful stock. Ask your butcher for soup bones or shank bones; they are inexpensive and easy to find.

4 pounds beef bones
2 carrots, peeled and quartered
2 stalks celery, quartered
¼ cup white-wine vinegar
2 bay leaves
1 tablespoon salt (optional)
4 quarts cold water

1. Combine the bones, carrots, celery, vinegar, bay leaves, and salt, if using, in a large stockpot or a 6-quart slow cooker. Add the water to cover. If using a stockpot, bring the mixture to a boil over high heat, reduce the heat to low, and simmer, stirring occasionally, for at least 8 hours (you can let it simmer for up to 24 hours or even longer if desired). If using a slow cooker, cover and cook on low for at least 12 hours.

2. Remove from the heat and let cool. Strain the broth through a fine-meshed sieve, discarding the solids, into glass jars. Let cool to room temperature. Cover the jars and refrigerate for up to a week, or freeze for up to 3 months.

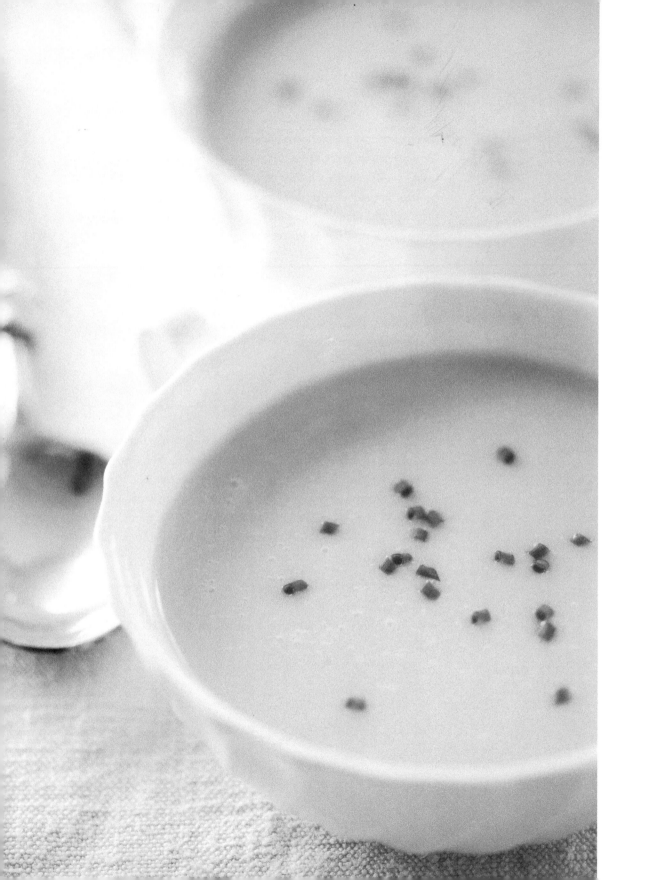

Creamy Potato Soup

SERVES 4

PREP TIME: 5 MINUTES

COOK TIME: 15 MINUTES

Cooking Tip: This soup can be made in a slow cooker instead of on the stovetop. Just put all of the ingredients into the slow cooker, cover, and cook on low for 6 hours or on high for 4 hours. Purée the soup just before serving.

PER SERVING

Calories: 340
Protein: 13g
Total Fat: 6g
Saturated Fat: 1g
Carbohydrates: 60g
Fiber: 4g
Sodium: 1778mg

This golden soup is rich and creamy without any dairy. Its flavor is simple yet satisfying. For a more adventurous soup, replace the nutmeg with diced, roasted green chiles, or top it with a garnish of crumbled bacon.

1 tablespoon olive oil
4 or 5 large Yukon Gold potatoes, peeled and diced
6 cups homemade (onion- and garlic-free) vegetable or chicken broth
1 cup unsweetened boxed coconut milk or rice milk
1 teaspoon salt
⅛ teaspoon ground nutmeg

1. In a stockpot over medium heat, heat the olive oil. Add the potatoes and cook, stirring, until they just begin to soften and color, for about 5 minutes.

2. Add the broth, cover, and simmer until the potatoes are tender, for about 10 minutes.

3. Stir in the coconut milk or rice milk and simmer for another few minutes until heated through.

4. Using an immersion blender or in batches in a countertop blender, purée the soup until smooth. Add the salt and nutmeg. Reheat if needed. Serve hot.

Banana-Rice Milk Smoothie

SERVES 2

PREP TIME: 5 MINUTES

COOK TIME: NONE

Substitution Tip: Coconut and banana is a sublime flavor combination, so feel free to substitute coconut milk for the rice milk.

PER SERVING

Calories: 173
Protein: 2g
Total Fat: 2g
Saturated Fat: 0g
Carbohydrates: 42g
Fiber: 9g
Sodium: 215mg

Bananas and rice are bland diet mainstays. Here they're combined in a soothing, nourishing, and filling smoothie. A bit of brown sugar sweetens things up, while a hint of vanilla extract rounds out the flavor.

2 cups unsweetened rice milk
2 ripe bananas
1 to 2 tablespoons brown sugar
1 teaspoon vanilla extract
Pinch of salt
4 to 6 ice cubes

Combine all of the ingredients in a blender and blend on high speed until smooth. Serve immediately.

Berry and Chia Seed Smoothie

SERVES 2

PREP TIME: 5 MINUTES, PLUS 10 MINUTES TO SOAK CHIA SEEDS

COOK TIME: NONE

Ingredient Tip: Frozen berries are a great substitute for fresh ones in smoothies. Feel free to use them whenever fresh berries are unavailable or out of season. You can also freeze surplus fresh berries in season and use as needed.

PER SERVING

Calories: 220
Protein: 3g
Total Fat: 6g
Saturated Fat: 0g
Carbohydrates: 42g
Fiber: 6g
Sodium: 81mg

Made with sweet blueberries and strawberries, this quick and easy smoothie provides a great weekday breakfast or a quick anytime snack. Chia seeds add thickness and body as well as a good dose of protein.

2 tablespoons chia seeds
2 cups unsweetened rice milk, divided
1 cup blueberries
1 cup strawberries
1 teaspoon vanilla extract

1. Place the chia seeds in a small bowl and pour ½ cup of the rice milk over them. Let the mixture sit for at least 10 minutes.

2. Transfer the chia seed mixture to a blender, add the remaining rice milk, blueberries, strawberries, and vanilla, and blend on high speed until smooth. Serve immediately.

Simple Rice Porridge

PREP TIME: 5 MINUTES

COOK TIME: 1 HOUR,
30 MINUTES

Substitution Tip: For additional flavor and added nutrition, substitute vegetable, chicken, or beef broth for the water. Depending on the saltiness of your broth, you may want to omit the salt.

PER SERVING

Calories: 113
Protein: 2g
Total Fat: 0g
Saturated Fat: 0g
Carbohydrates: 25g
Fiber: 0g
Sodium: 789mg

Rice porridge, also called juk *or* congee, *is a traditional Chinese breakfast food. In Chinese kitchens, it is usually served with savory side dishes or garnishes such as ginger, sesame oil, soy sauce, and sliced scallions, as well as with cooked chicken, or cooked or pickled vegetables. Feel free to add garnishes for additional flavor or nutrition, or just eat it as is for a filling and soothing meal.*

1 cup long-grain white rice, well rinsed
10 cups water
2 teaspoons salt (optional)

In a large, heavy saucepan, combine the rice, water, and salt, if using, and bring to a boil over high heat. Lower the heat to medium-low, cover, and simmer, stirring occasionally, for about 1½ hours, until the rice is very soft and the mixture is thick.

Coconut-Banana Oatmeal

SERVES 2

PREP TIME: 2 MINUTES

COOK TIME: 12 MINUTES

Ingredient Tip: If you have celiac disease or are on a very strict gluten-free diet, be sure to use certified gluten-free oats.

PER SERVING

Calories: 346
Protein: 5.1g
Total Fat: 13.8g
Saturated Fat: 11g
Carbohydrates: 55.9g
Fiber: 5.1g
Sodium: 21.9mg

Oatmeal flavored with creamy coconut milk and sweet bananas makes a soothing and nourishing breakfast. Add a bit of brown sugar if you prefer more sweetness, or add fresh fruits, like blueberries or sliced strawberries.

1¾ cups water
½ cup rolled oats
½ cup canned coconut milk
2 ripe bananas, peeled and cut into ¼-inch-thick slices
2 tablespoons brown sugar (optional)

1. In a saucepan, combine the water, oats, coconut milk, and banana and bring to a simmer over medium-high heat. Reduce the heat to medium-low and cook, uncovered, for about 10 minutes, until the liquid has been absorbed and the oats are tender.

2. To serve, spoon into bowls and top with brown sugar if desired.

Oven-Baked Polenta Porridge with Strawberries

SERVES 4

PREP TIME: 5 MINUTES

COOK TIME: 1 HOUR

Substitution Tip: Feel free to substitute a vegan butter substitute, such as Earth Balance, for the coconut oil.

PER SERVING

Calories: 535
Protein: 6g
Total Fat: 30g
Saturated Fat: 25g
Carbohydrates: 65g
Fiber: 0g
Sodium: 170mg

Polenta is usually topped with savory but heavy meat-based sauces, like Bolognese, but when baked with creamy coconut milk and a touch of maple syrup and topped with fresh strawberries, it makes a delightful breakfast porridge. For a savory dish that's similarly easy to digest, just leave out the maple syrup and top with any flavorful sauce of your choice.

1½ tablespoons coconut oil, plus more for preparing the baking dish
2 cups water
1 (14-ounce) can light coconut milk
1½ cups polenta
2 tablespoons maple syrup
¼ teaspoon salt
1 pint strawberries, sliced

1. Preheat the oven to 350°F.

2. Grease a 9-by-13-inch baking dish with coconut oil. In the prepared dish, stir together the 1½ tablespoons of coconut oil, water, coconut milk, polenta, maple syrup, and salt. Bake, uncovered, for 60 minutes.

3. To serve, spoon into serving bowls and top with strawberries.

Risotto and Vegetable Soup

SERVES 4

PREP TIME: 5 MINUTES

COOK TIME: 35 MINUTES

Substitution Tip: For even more nutrition, plus added flavor, try using Roasted-Vegetable Broth (page 38) or Chicken-Bone Broth (page 40) in place of regular vegetable broth.

PER SERVING

Calories: 286
Protein: 11g
Total Fat: 6g
Saturated Fat: 1g
Carbohydrates: 46g
Fiber: 3g
Sodium: 1763mg

Like a soupy risotto, this rice and veggie soup is a filling and satisfying meal on its own. If you're feeling up to it, add extra substance with chunks of cooked chicken, a poached egg, or a handful of freshly grated Parmesan cheese.

1 tablespoon olive oil
3 medium carrots, diced
1 cup Arborio rice
6 cups homemade (onion- and garlic-free) vegetable broth
1 bay leaf
1 teaspoon salt
1 cup frozen green beans

1. Heat the oil in a medium stockpot over medium heat.

2. Add the carrots. Reduce the heat and cook, stirring occasionally, until they have softened, for about 10 minutes.

3. Add the rice to the pot and stir well, until each grain is coated with oil. Add the broth, bay leaf, and salt and bring just to a boil over medium-high heat. Reduce the heat, cover, and simmer for about 20 minutes, until the rice is tender and cooked through.

4. Stir in the green beans and cook, stirring occasionally, for another 5 minutes or so, until the beans are tender. Serve hot.

Carrot Purée

SERVES 4

PREP TIME: 5 MINUTES

COOK TIME: 15 MINUTES

Substitution Tip: For a vegan and dairy-free version, use vegetable broth and substitute full-fat coconut milk for the cream.

PER SERVING

Calories: 84
Protein: 2g
Total Fat: 4g
Saturated Fat: 3g
Carbohydrates: 10g
Fiber: 2g
Sodium: 501mg

Bright-orange carrots are simmered in broth and puréed with a touch of heavy cream for a sublime side dish that is perfect alongside roasted meat or fish. This is one of those dishes that are surprisingly simple to make and also unexpectedly delicious. Even your kids will love it!

⅔ cup homemade (onion- and garlic-free) vegetable or
  chicken broth
6 medium carrots, halved lengthwise and cut into
  ½-inch pieces
½ teaspoon salt
3 tablespoons heavy cream
freshly ground black pepper

1. In a medium saucepan, heat the broth to a simmer over medium heat. Reduce the heat, add the carrots and salt, cover, and simmer for about 12 minutes, until the carrots are very tender.

2. Transfer the mixture to a food processor or blender, add the cream, and purée until smooth. Season with black pepper and serve immediately.

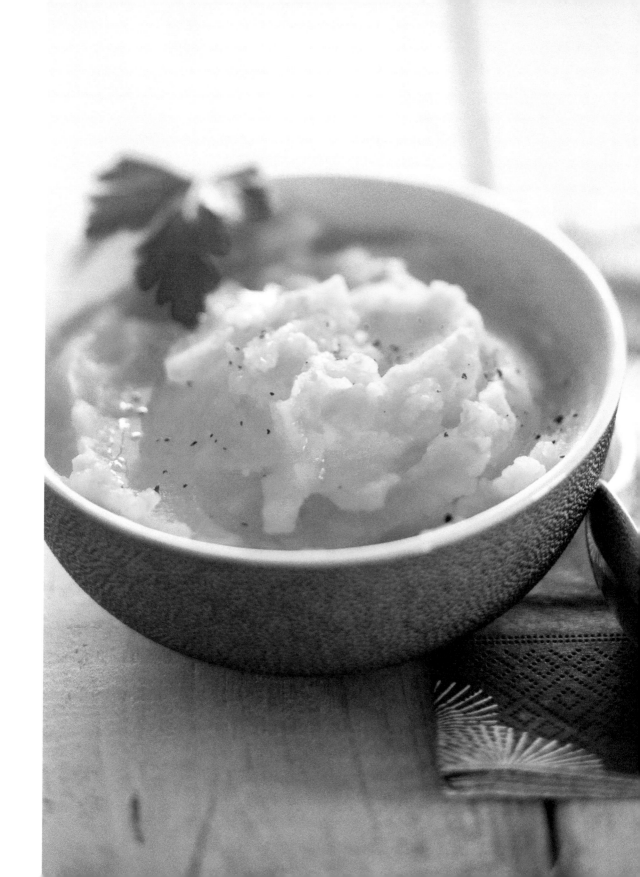

Egg-Drop Soup

SERVES 4

PREP TIME: 10 MINUTES

COOK TIME: 25 MINUTES

Substitution Tip: For an egg-free version of this soup, simply omit the eggs and add hot, cooked rice noodles, such as Thai rice sticks, just before serving.

PER SERVING

Calories: 279
Protein: 38g
Total Fat: 10g
Saturated Fat: 2g
Carbohydrates: 8g
Fiber: 1g
Sodium: 1890mg

This simmering broth with aromatic herbs, including ginger, peppercorns, cloves, and cinnamon, imparts a deep, rich flavor. If desired, garnish the soup with sesame oil, Garlic Oil (page 202), or other flavorings.

6 cups homemade (onion- and garlic-free) chicken or vegetable broth
1 teaspoon salt
½-inch piece of fresh ginger, peeled and cut into thin rounds
½ teaspoon peppercorns
6 whole cloves
1 cinnamon stick
2 tablespoons cornstarch, divided
4 large eggs
2 cups cooked, shredded chicken, warmed
2 scallions (green parts only), thinly sliced

1. In a stockpot or saucepan, combine the broth, salt, ginger, peppercorns, cloves, and cinnamon and heat to a simmer over medium-high heat. Reduce the heat to prevent the mixture from boiling and simmer for 15 minutes. Strain the solids out of the broth and discard them.

2. In a small bowl, whisk together ¼ cup of the stock and 1 tablespoon plus 1½ teaspoons of the cornstarch. Bring the stock in the pot back to a vigorous simmer, stir in the cornstarch mixture, and cook, stirring, for about 2 minutes, until the broth thickens.

3. In a small bowl, whisk the eggs with the remaining 1½ teaspoons cornstarch. With the soup at a simmer, gently drizzle the eggs into the soup and whisk the soup gently. Let it simmer for another 30 seconds or so, until the eggs are cooked through. Serve immediately, garnished with the shredded chicken and scallions.

Ginger-Steamed Chicken Breast

SERVES 4

PREP TIME: 5 MINUTES

COOK TIME: 10 MINUTES

Ingredient Tip: Cooking chicken on the bone maintains maximum flavor but takes a bit longer. Feel free to substitute bone-in chicken breasts, cooking them for an additional 5 minutes or so. You can also leave the skin on, if you like, which will add additional flavor and moisture, as well as some additional fat.

PER SERVING

Calories: 328
Protein: 49g
Total Fat: 13g
Saturated Fat: 4g
Carbohydrates: 1g
Fiber: 0g
Sodium: 728mg

Steaming chicken breast in a bath of moist heat keeps it from drying out and doesn't require the use of any added fat, making this a great cooking method when you are dealing with painful digestive symptoms that may be exacerbated by fatty foods. Ginger adds flavor and also serves as a digestive aid, stimulating the release of enzymes that help your body break down and absorb foods. Serve this chicken plain or over Simple Rice Porridge (page 46) or steamed rice, or dice it for tossing into salads, noodles, or other dishes.

4 boneless, skinless chicken-breast halves
1 teaspoon salt
1 tablespoon minced ginger

1. Season the chicken breasts on all sides with the salt. Place them in a single layer in a steamer basket set over a pot of simmering water. Sprinkle the minced ginger over the chicken.

2. Cover the pot and cook for 8 to 10 minutes, until the chicken is cooked through.

Vanilla Pudding

SERVES 4

PREP TIME: 5 MINUTES,
PLUS 2 HOURS TO CHILL

COOK TIME: 5 MINUTES

Substitution Tip: You can substitute lactose-free milk or coconut milk for the rice milk, if desired.

PER SERVING

Calories: 119
Protein: 1g
Total Fat: 1g
Saturated Fat: 0g
Carbohydrates: 27g
Fiber: 3g
Sodium: 217mg

Creamy vanilla pudding is the ultimate comfort food. This dairy-free version is easy to make, requiring just a few minutes of preparation and cooking time. Serve it topped with sliced bananas or strawberries, or make it festive by layering it with fruit in a parfait.

2 cups unsweetened rice milk
⅓ cup cornstarch
2 tablespoons maple syrup
¼ teaspoon salt
1 tablespoon vanilla extract

1. In a medium saucepan, combine the rice milk, cornstarch, maple syrup, and salt, whisking until smooth. Bring the mixture to a boil over medium heat, stirring constantly, and cook until it thickens, for about 2 to 3 minutes more. Remove from the heat and stir in the vanilla.

2. Cover and chill for at least 2 hours.

3. Transfer the mixture to a blender or food processor and process until smooth. Serve immediately.

Coconut Rice Pudding

SERVES 4

PREP TIME: 5 MINUTES

COOK TIME: 60 MINUTES

Cooking Tip: Using leftover cooked rice saves time and effort. Plan ahead by making extra rice for dinner one night, and remember not to salt it before or during cooking.

PER SERVING

Calories: 308
Protein: 2.7g
Total Fat: 8g
Saturated Fat: 0g
Carbohydrates: 53g
Fiber: 0.3g
Sodium: 209mg

This creamy rice pudding is made with coconut milk, which brings exotic flavor to this old-school dish. Sweetened with just a touch of brown sugar, it can be served on its own or topped with fresh fruit. Diced pineapple would provide a nice complement to the tropical flavor of coconut or, for a splash of color, try fresh blueberries or sliced strawberries.

¾ cup short- or medium-grain white rice
1¼ cups water
1½ cups unsweetened rice milk
1 (14-ounce) can light coconut milk
¼ cup brown sugar
¼ teaspoon salt
1 teaspoon vanilla

1. In a medium saucepan, combine the rice with the water and bring to a boil over high heat. Reduce the heat to low, cover, and simmer until the rice is tender and the liquid has been absorbed, for about 20 minutes.

2. In a large saucepan, combine the rice, rice milk, coconut milk, sugar, and salt, and cook over medium heat, stirring often, until the mixture is thickened, for about 40 minutes. Stir in the vanilla and serve immediately.

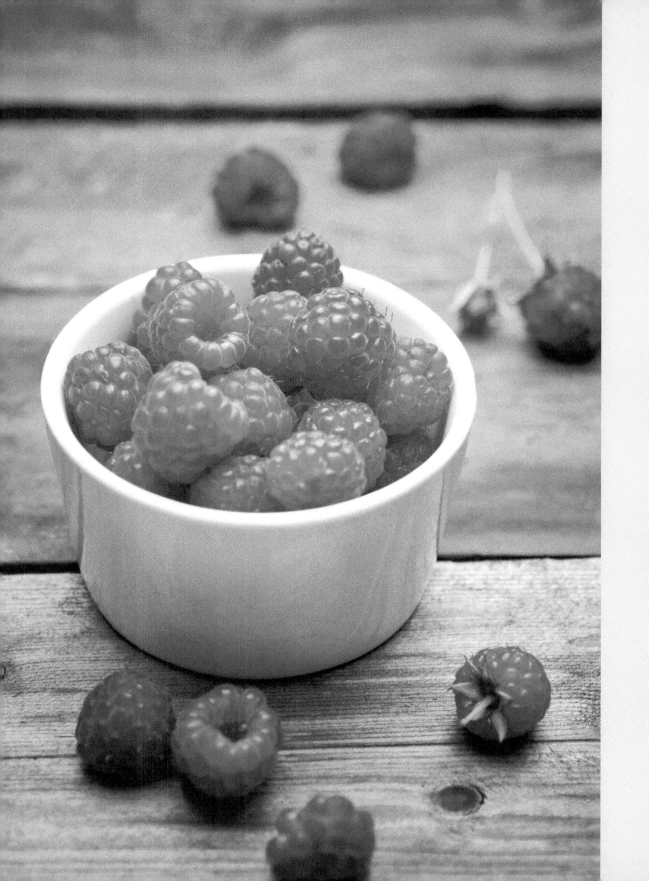

4

Breakfast and Brunch

Peanut Butter Granola

SERVES 4

PREP TIME: 5 MINUTES

COOK TIME: 10 MINUTES

Substitution Tip: If you can't eat nuts, substitute sunflower-seed butter for the peanut butter.

PER SERVING

Calories: 340
Protein: 12g
Total Fat: 19g
Saturated Fat: 3g
Carbohydrates: 36g
Fiber: 4g
Sodium: 79mg

This crispy, peanut buttery granola is simply irresistible in a bowl with (lactose-free or nondairy) milk or sprinkled over fruit or dairy-free ice cream. Start with this basic recipe and add other ingredients as the mood strikes. Shredded coconut, raisins, and sunflower seeds would all be tasty additions.

Coconut oil for preparing the baking sheet
¼ cup creamy peanut butter
¼ cup maple syrup
½ teaspoon cinnamon
½ teaspoon vanilla extract
1 cup gluten-free oats
½ cup pumpkin seeds
2 tablespoons sunflower seeds

1. Preheat the oven to 325°F.

2. Oil a large, rimmed baking sheet with coconut oil.

3. In the top of a double boiler set over simmering water, stir together the peanut butter and maple syrup until the peanut butter melts and the mixture is well combined, for about 2 minutes. Stir in the cinnamon and vanilla.

4. In a medium bowl, combine the peanut butter mixture with the oats, pumpkin seeds, and sunflower seeds and stir until the oats and seeds are well coated.

5. Spread the oat mixture onto the prepared baking sheet and bake in the preheated oven for about 8 minutes, until lightly browned. Remove from the oven and let the granola cool. It will become crisp as it cools. Serve at room temperature.

Chia Seed Carrot Cake Pudding

SERVES 2

PREP TIME: 5 MINUTES,
PLUS OVERNIGHT TO CHILL

COOK TIME: NONE

Substitution Tip: You can replace the rice milk with lactose-free milk or any nondairy milk substitute you like.

PER SERVING

Calories: 135
Protein: 3g
Total Fat: 5g
Saturated Fat: 0g
Carbohydrates: 26g
Fiber: 8g
Sodium: 88mg

Soaking the chia seeds overnight transforms them into a simple tapioca-like breakfast pudding. This version includes all the spicy flavors of your favorite carrot cake but with none of the dairy, gluten, or eggs you'd find in a cake. Even better, it's sweetened with just a touch of maple syrup.

¾ cup unsweetened rice milk
½ cup chopped carrots
3 tablespoons chia seeds, divided
2 tablespoons maple syrup
½ teaspoon vanilla
½ teaspoon cinnamon
¼ teaspoon ground ginger
⅛ teaspoon ground cloves
Pinch nutmeg

1. Place the rice milk, carrots, 2 tablespoons of the chia seeds, maple syrup, vanilla, cinnamon, ginger, cloves, and nutmeg in a blender and blend until smooth. Add the remaining tablespoon of chia seeds and pulse just to incorporate.

2. Pour the mixture into two custard cups or bowls, cover, and refrigerate overnight. Serve chilled.

Orange-Scented Overnight Oatmeal

SERVES 4

PREP TIME: 5 MINUTES,
PLUS OVERNIGHT TO SOAK

COOK TIME: NONE

Substitution Tip: For a
dairy-free version of this
dish, substitute rice milk
or coconut milk for the
lactose-free milk.

PER SERVING

Calories: 231
Protein: 10g
Total Fat: 4g
Saturated Fat: 1g
Carbohydrates: 39g
Fiber: 6g
Sodium: 35mg

Overnight oats make a welcome breakfast on busy mornings. Mix the ingredients the night before, and your breakfast will be ready before you even get out of bed. This version is sweetened with orange juice and maple syrup.

1 cup gluten-free rolled oats
1¼ cups lactose-free milk, divided
Juice of ½ orange
½ tablespoon chia seeds
1 tablespoon maple syrup, divided
¼ teaspoon cinnamon
½ teaspoon vanilla extract
¼ teaspoon orange extract
⅛ teaspoon ground ginger

1. In a medium bowl, stir together the oats, 1 cup of the milk, orange juice, chia seeds, half of the maple syrup, cinnamon, vanilla and orange extracts, and ginger. Cover and refrigerate overnight.

2. To serve, stir in the remaining maple syrup, and serve chilled or warmed.

Everything-Free Pancakes

SERVES 4

PREP TIME: 5 MINUTES,
PLUS 3 MINUTES TO SOAK
THE CHIA-SEED MEAL

COOK TIME: 10 MINUTES

Ingredient Tip: Be sure
to use a gluten-free
flour that is made with
low-FODMAP grains and
starches, such as King
Arthur's.

PER SERVING

Calories: 528
Protein: 7g
Total Fat: 19g
Saturated Fat: 15g
Carbohydrates: 82g
Fiber: 3g
Sodium: 472mg

These pancakes are free of all common allergens, including gluten, eggs, dairy, soy, and nuts, but they are packed with flavor. Serve them topped with sliced bananas or fresh berries and a drizzle of maple syrup. A dollop of lightly sweetened whipped cream would make a delightful finishing touch.

⅓ cup warm water

2 tablespoons chia-seed meal

¼ cup maple syrup

5 tablespoons coconut oil, melted, divided

2 teaspoons vanilla extract

2 cups gluten-free flour (see Ingredient Tip)

½ teaspoon salt

¾ teaspoon baking powder

½ teaspoon baking soda

1. In a large bowl, combine the warm water and chia-seed meal. Let it sit for about 3 minutes, until the mixture is thickened. Stir in the maple syrup, 3 tablespoons of the coconut oil, vanilla extract, and gluten-free flour, and whisk to combine. Add the salt, baking powder, and baking soda, and whisk to incorporate.

2. Heat 1 tablespoon of the coconut oil in a large skillet over medium-high heat.

3. Ladle the batter, ¼ cup at a time, into the heated skillet. Cook until bubbles appear on the tops of the pancakes, about 2 to 3 minutes. Flip over and cook until the second side is golden brown, about 1 to 2 minutes more. Repeat with the remaining batter, adding more oil to the pan as needed. Serve hot, topped with fresh fruit, if desired.

Ginger-Berry Rice Milk Smoothie

SERVES 2

PREP TIME: 5 MINUTES

COOK TIME: NONE

Substitution Tip: You can substitute coconut milk or another nondairy milk for the rice milk if desired.

PER SERVING

Calories: 162
Protein: 2g
Total Fat: 2g
Saturated Fat: 0g
Carbohydrates: 37g
Fiber: 8g
Sodium 71mg

Smoothies make a great, healthy, quick, and portable breakfast. This one includes digestive system-soothing fresh ginger. You can use any berries you like: strawberries, blueberries, raspberries, or a combination.

2 cups frozen strawberries, blueberries, or raspberries
1 cup unsweetened rice milk
2 tablespoons maple syrup
2 teaspoons finely grated fresh ginger
2 teaspoons lemon juice

Place all of the ingredients in a blender and blend until smooth. Serve immediately.

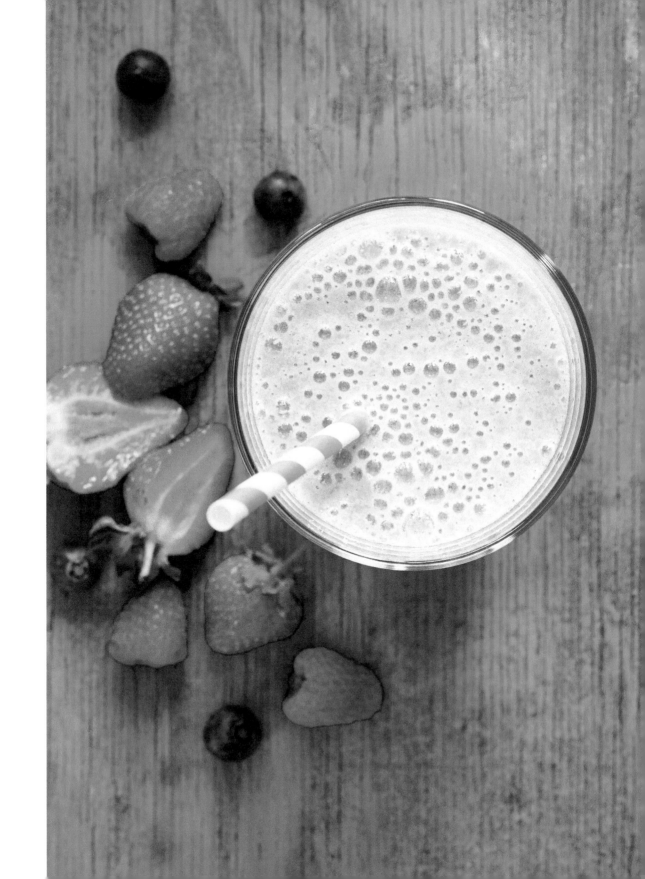

Strawberry-Kiwi Smoothie with Chia Seeds

PREP TIME: 5 MINUTES

COOK TIME: NONE

Substitution Tip:
If desired, substitute blueberries, raspberries, or a combination of both.

PER SERVING

Calories: 294
Protein: 4g
Total Fat: 5g
Saturated Fat: 0g
Carbohydrates: 63g
Fiber: 8g
Sodium: 43mg

This smoothie takes merely a few minutes to prepare but is packed with nutrition and flavor. Chia seeds at once thicken it and give it a healthy boost of protein.

¾ **cup orange juice**
¾ **cup unsweetened rice milk**
1 ripe banana, peeled and sliced
2 kiwifruit, peeled and sliced
10 frozen strawberries
2 tablespoons maple syrup
2 tablespoons chia seeds

Place all of the ingredients in a blender and blend until smooth. Serve immediately.

Quinoa Breakfast Bowl with Basil "Hollandaise" Sauce

SERVES 4

PREP TIME: 10 MINUTES

COOK TIME: 15 MINUTES

Substitution Tip: For added flavor, cook the quinoa in vegetable or chicken broth instead of water. Depending on the saltiness of your broth, you may want to omit the salt.

PER SERVING

Calories: 415
Protein: 9g
Total Fat: 28g
Saturated Fat: 3g
Carbohydrates: 36g
Fiber: 6g
Sodium: 605mg

Quinoa is a favorite grain among those who eschew gluten. Not only is it delicious and a great base for a variety of sauces and toppings, but it is also full of protein. Enjoy this tasty breakfast bowl as is, or top it with a poached or fried egg.

1 cup uncooked quinoa
12 ounces green beans, trimmed and cut into 1-inch pieces
1½ cups water
½ teaspoon salt
Basil "Hollandaise" Sauce (page 211)

1. In a medium saucepan, stir together the quinoa, green beans, water, and salt. Bring to a boil over medium-high heat. Reduce the heat to low, cover, and simmer for about 15 minutes, until the quinoa is tender.

2. To serve, spoon the quinoa mixture into bowls and drizzle the sauce over the top.

Oven-Baked Zucchini and Carrot Fritters with Ginger-Lime Sauce

SERVES 4

PREP TIME: 10 MINUTES,
PLUS 15 MINUTES TO DRAIN
THE ZUCCHINI

COOK TIME: 40 MINUTES

Substitution Tip: To make this an egg-free recipe, try using a chia-seed egg replacer: Grind 2 tablespoons white chia-seed meal in a food processor or spice grinder, and mix with 6 tablespoons warm water. Let the mixture stand for 5 to 10 minutes, until it thickens to the consistency of raw eggs.

PER SERVING

Calories: 296
Protein: 8g
Total Fat: 18g
Saturated Fat: 14g
Carbohydrates: 30g
Fiber: 5g
Sodium: 88mg

These veggie fritters are a breeze to prepare for a crowd, because they're baked en masse in the oven. The sauce is simple to whip up in a blender and makes the dish feel brunch worthy.

Oil for preparing the baking sheet
2 large zucchini
1 teaspoon salt
2 large carrots
1 cup chopped cilantro, plus additional for garnish
2 eggs, lightly beaten
1 tablespoon gluten-free, onion- and garlic-free curry powder
2 teaspoons gluten-free, onion- and garlic-free chili powder
2 teaspoons cumin
½ cup brown-rice flour
1 cup coconut milk
2 tablespoons lemon juice
1 tablespoon lime juice
1 teaspoon cornstarch
1 teaspoon sugar
¾ teaspoon ground ginger

1. Preheat the oven to 400°F.

2. Line a large baking sheet with parchment paper and lightly oil the parchment.

3. In a food processor, pulse the zucchini to chop it finely. Transfer the chopped zucchini to a colander set over the sink and sprinkle generously with salt. Let sit for about 15 minutes.

4. Finely chop the carrots and cilantro in the food processor, then combine with the zucchini in a large mixing bowl. Add the eggs, curry powder, chili powder, and cumin. Stir to mix.

5. Add the flour, ¼ cup at a time, stirring to incorporate it.

6. Drop the batter onto the prepared baking sheet by heaping tablespoons, flattening the fritters with the back of the spoon.

7. Bake in the preheated oven for 25 minutes. Turn the fritters over and continue to bake for another 15 to 20 minutes, until the fritters are crisp and golden brown.

8. While the fritters are in the oven, make the sauce. In a small bowl, stir together the coconut milk, lemon juice, lime juice, cornstarch, sugar, and ginger.

9. Serve the fritters hot, with a drizzle of the sauce and a sprinkling of cilantro.

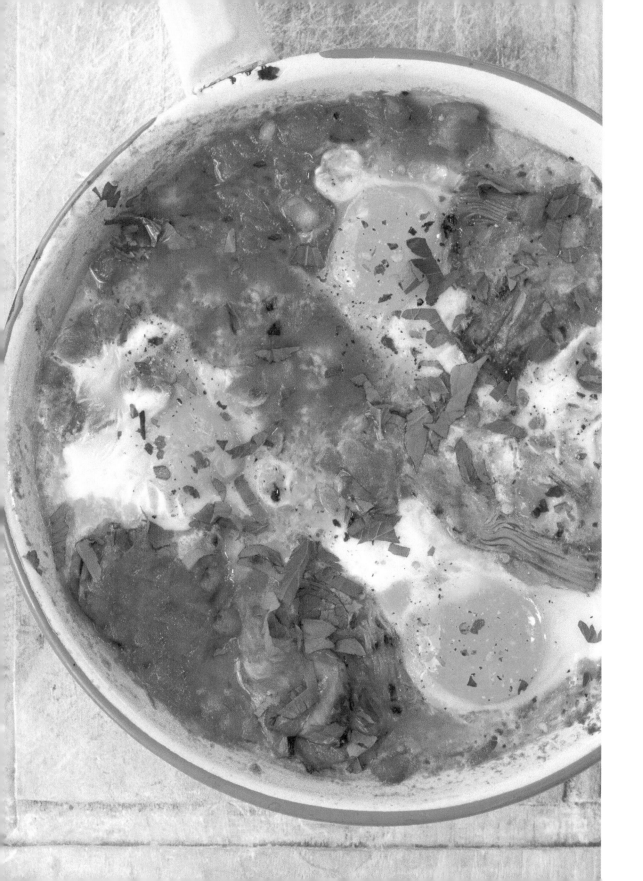

Breakfast Ratatouille with Poached Eggs

SERVES 4

PREP TIME: 15 MINUTES

COOK TIME: 40 MINUTES

Substitution Tip: For a dairy- and egg-free version, substitute coconut oil or olive oil for the butter, omit the eggs and cheese, and serve the vegetables over cooked quinoa.

PER SERVING

Calories: 292
Protein: 21g
Total Fat: 15g
Saturated Fat: 7g
Carbohydrates: 24g
Fiber: 10g
Sodium: 819mg

This Provence-style summer vegetable stew makes a great brunch dish topped with poached eggs. The stew improves with time, so go ahead and make it the day before. Then simply reheat it and poach the eggs just before serving. For extra flavor, add a drizzle of Garlic Oil (page 202) just before serving.

2 tablespoons butter
1 medium eggplant, diced
4 medium tomatoes, peeled, seeded, and diced
1 red bell pepper, diced
1 green bell pepper, diced
2 medium zucchini, diced
½ cup halved artichoke hearts
1 jalapeño, diced
2 tablespoons chopped fresh thyme
1 tablespoon chopped fresh oregano
¼ cup chopped parsley
**½ cup homemade (onion- and garlic-free) chicken or
  vegetable broth**
1 teaspoon salt
½ teaspoon freshly ground pepper
4 eggs
2 ounces freshly grated Parmesan cheese

1. Heat the butter in a large skillet over medium-high heat. Add the eggplant and cook, stirring occasionally, for about 10 minutes, until the eggplant is tender. Add the tomatoes and cook for about 5 minutes, until the tomatoes have begun to break down.

2. Add the bell peppers, zucchini, artichoke hearts, jalapeño, thyme, oregano, and parsley. Stir to mix. Add the broth, salt, and pepper, and bring to a boil. Cover, reduce the heat to low, and simmer for about 20 minutes, until the liquid has evaporated and the vegetables are tender. ▶

3. While the vegetables are cooking, poach the eggs. Bring a pan of water about 3 inches deep to a boil over high heat. Reduce the heat to low, carefully break the eggs into the water, and simmer for 4 minutes.

4. To serve, ladle the vegetable mixture into 4 serving bowls, top each with a poached egg, and sprinkle the cheese over the top. Serve hot.

Eggplant Bacon

SERVES 4

PREP TIME: 5 MINUTES,
PLUS 30 MINUTES
TO MARINATE

COOK TIME: 10 MINUTES

Substitution Tip: If you
are sensitive to soy,
substitute coconut
aminos for the soy sauce.

PER SERVING

Calories: 151
Protein: 1g
Total Fat: 10g
Saturated Fat: 1g
Carbohydrates: 15g
Fiber: 5g
Sodium: 52mg

Like regular bacon, eggplant bacon adds a crisp crunch and salty umami flavor to everything from salads to sandwiches or burgers. In preparing it, the eggplant is sliced thinly and marinated in soy sauce and other flavorings, then cooked in a skillet until crispy. This dish makes an excellent accompaniment to eggs, tucked into a vegetarian BLT, or crumbled and sprinkled over any food that needs a little crunch or extra flavor.

¼ cup gluten-free soy sauce
¼ cup rice vinegar
2 tablespoons plus 2 teaspoons olive oil, divided
2 tablespoons maple syrup
2 teaspoons liquid smoke
1 medium eggplant, sliced lengthwise into ¼-inch slabs

1. In a medium bowl, combine the soy sauce, vinegar, 2 tablespoons of the olive oil, maple syrup, and liquid smoke.

2. Add the eggplant, toss to coat, and let marinate for 30 minutes, tossing occasionally.

3. Heat the remaining 2 teaspoons of olive oil in a large skillet over medium-high heat. Drain the eggplant slices, reserving the marinade, and cook in a single layer, in batches if needed, for about 5 minutes, until browned on the bottom. Add half of the reserved marinade to the pan (or one-quarter if you are cooking the eggplant in two batches) and cook for another minute, until the liquid has evaporated. Turn the eggplant slices over and cook for another 5 minutes or so, until the second side is browned. Add the remaining marinade (or half of the remaining marinade if cooking two batches) and cook until the liquid has evaporated, for another minute.

Gluten-Free Eggs Benedict

SERVES 4

PREP TIME: 10 MINUTES

COOK TIME: 30 MINUTES

Substitution Tip: For an egg-free version of this recipe, substitute Basil "Hollandaise" Sauce (page 211) for the traditional Hollandaise sauce here. You can also substitute Eggplant Bacon (page 71) for a veggie version.

PER SERVING

Calories: 550
Protein: 26g
Total Fat: 28g
Saturated Fat: 12g
Carbohydrates: 49g
Fiber: 2g
Sodium: 1231mg

Eggs Benedict is a decadent brunch dish that's usually off limits to those who maintain a gluten-free diet, but here the English muffins are replaced with rounds of crisp oven-baked polenta. The rest of the dish maintains the perfection of the original: browned Canadian bacon or ham, lemony Hollandaise sauce, and plump poached eggs.

Olive oil for preparing the pan and brushing the polenta slices
8 (½-inch-thick) slices precooked polenta (from an 18-ounce tube)
8 eggs
8 slices ham or Canadian bacon

FOR THE SAUCE
1 large egg yolk
1½ teaspoons lemon juice
½ teaspoon salt
4 tablespoons (½ stick) unsalted butter, melted

1. Preheat the oven to 375°F.

2. Oil a large baking sheet, arrange the polenta slices on the prepared sheet, and brush the tops with olive oil. Bake the polenta rounds in the preheated oven for 18 to 20 minutes, until they are golden brown and crisp.

3. Meanwhile, make the sauce. In a blender, add the egg yolk, lemon juice, and salt, and blend for about 5 seconds, until just combined.

4. Set the blender to high, and add the butter to the yolk mixture in a thin stream until the sauce is thick and smooth, which will happen almost immediately. If the sauce thickens too much, add 1 or 2 teaspoons of warm water.

5. To poach the eggs, bring a pan of water about 3 inches deep to a boil over high heat. Reduce the heat to low, carefully break the eggs into the water, and simmer for 4 minutes.

6. While the eggs cook, heat a large skillet over medium-high heat. Add the ham or Canadian bacon slices in a single layer and cook until they begin to brown, for about 3 minutes. Turn over and cook on the other side until hot and just beginning to brown, for about 1 minute.

7. To serve, arrange 2 polenta slices on each of 4 serving plates. Top each round with a slice of ham or Canadian bacon, a poached egg, and a drizzle of the Hollandaise sauce. Serve immediately.

Potato Pancakes

SERVES 4

PREP TIME: 10 MINUTES

COOK TIME: 10 MINUTES

Substitution Tip: To make this an egg-free recipe, try using a chia-seed egg replacer. Grind 2 tablespoons white chia-seed meal in a food processor or spice grinder, and mix with 6 tablespoons warm water. Let the mixture stand for 5 to 10 minutes until it thickens to the consistency of raw eggs.

PER SERVING

Calories: 169
Protein: 6g
Total Fat: 3g
Saturated Fat: 2g
Carbohydrates: 30g
Fiber: 4g
Sodium: 332mg

These crispy, golden-brown potato patties make a terrific substitute for toast as a platform for fried or poached eggs. If you're feeling decadent, you might even top them with Basil "Hollandaise" Sauce (page 211).

3 medium potatoes, peeled and quartered
2 eggs
2 tablespoons rice flour
½ teaspoon salt
¼ teaspoon freshly ground pepper
2 tablespoons coconut or grapeseed oil

1. In a blender or food processor, pulse the potatoes until they are finely chopped.

2. In a medium bowl, whisk the eggs, and then add the flour, salt, pepper, and the finely chopped potatoes, and stir to mix well.

3. Heat the oil in a large skillet over medium-high heat. Add the potato mixture about ¼ cup at a time, using the back of a spoon or scoop to flatten into pancakes about 3 inches in diameter. Cook for 3 to 4 minutes per side, until the pancakes are golden brown and crisp. Serve hot.

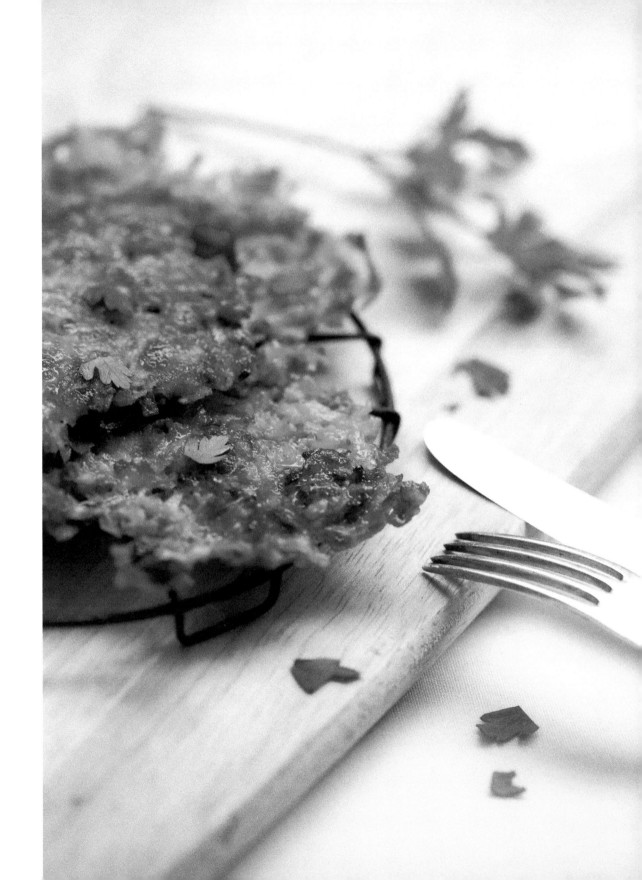

Huevos Rancheros

SERVES 4

PREP TIME: 10 MINUTES

COOK TIME: 20 MINUTES

Substitution Tip: For an egg-free version of this dish, replace the eggs with 1 cup of canned chickpeas along with the zucchini.

PER SERVING

Calories: 257
Protein: 10g
Total Fat: 13g
Saturated Fat: 4g
Carbohydrates: 29g
Fiber: 5g
Sodium: 695mg

Huevos rancheros is a breakfast classic: hot corn tortillas topped with fried eggs and smothered in a spicy tomato sauce. If you like, top it with diced avocado or pickled jalapeños for an extra punch of Latin flavor.

8 small corn tortillas
1 tablespoon butter
4 eggs
2 tablespoons chopped cilantro

FOR THE SAUCE
1 tablespoon olive oil
1 zucchini, diced
1 red, yellow, or green bell pepper, cored, seeded, diced
2 chopped jalapeños or 2 tablespoons roasted green chiles
2 plum tomatoes, peeled, seeded, and diced
1 teaspoon salt
½ teaspoon ground cumin
½ teaspoon gluten-free, onion- and garlic-free chili powder
½ teaspoon dried oregano
1 tablespoon Garlic Oil (page 202)

1. Preheat the oven to 400°F.

2. Wrap the tortillas in aluminum foil and bake in the preheated oven for about 10 minutes.

3. While the tortillas are heating, make the sauce. Heat the olive oil in a large skillet over medium-high heat. Add the zucchini, bell pepper, and jalapeños. Cook, stirring frequently, until the vegetables are softened and beginning to brown, for about 5 minutes. Add the tomatoes along with the salt, cumin, chili powder, and oregano. Cook, stirring, for about another 5 minutes, until the tomatoes break down and become saucy. Stir in the Garlic Oil.

4. Heat the butter in another large skillet over medium heat. Add the eggs and fry to desired doneness.

5. To serve, arrange 2 tortillas on each of 4 serving plates, and top with a fried egg and a generous serving of sauce. Garnish with cilantro and serve immediately.

Spicy Scrambled Chickpeas

SERVES 4

PREP TIME: 5 MINUTES

COOK TIME: 10 MINUTES

Substitution Tip: Feel free to add other vegetables as the season allows. Diced zucchini, eggplant, tomatoes, or green beans would all be welcome additions.

PER SERVING

Calories: 275
Protein: 12g
Total Fat: 10g
Saturated Fat: 1g
Carbohydrates: 26g
Fiber: 11g
Sodium: 547mg

A spicy scramble always makes for a satisfying breakfast, and this egg-free version of the classic scramble is no exception. Note that chickpeas contain moderate levels of FODMAPs, so stick to a single serving.

1 cup canned chickpeas, drained and rinsed
½ teaspoon paprika
½ teaspoon ground coriander
¼ teaspoon ground cumin
¼ teaspoon cayenne
¼ teaspoon freshly ground black pepper
2 tablespoons olive oil
1 red bell pepper, seeded and diced
1 yellow or orange bell pepper, seeded and diced
20 leaves Swiss chard, center ribs removed and leaves julienned
½ teaspoon salt
2 tablespoons chopped cilantro

1. In a bowl, combine the chickpeas with the paprika, coriander, cumin, cayenne, and pepper. Toss until chickpeas are evenly coated with the spices.

2. Heat the oil in a large skillet over high heat. Add the bell peppers and chard. Cook, stirring frequently, until the vegetables begin to soften and brown on the edges, for about 5 minutes.

3. Add the chickpea mixture, salt, and about 1 tablespoon of water. Cook, stirring, for 5 minutes, until the chickpeas are heated through and the water has evaporated. Serve immediately, garnished with cilantro.

Bacon and Sweet Potato Hash

SERVES 4

PREP TIME: 4 MINUTES

COOK TIME: 25 MINUTES

Substitution Tip: For a vegan version, omit the bacon in step 3 and substitute Eggplant Bacon (page 71), adding it at the end as a garnish.

PER SERVING

Calories: 267
Protein: 9g
Total Fat: 19g
Saturated Fat: 4g
Carbohydrates: 17g
Fiber: 4g
Sodium: 682mg

Tender sweet potatoes and crispy bacon come together in this satisfying and addictive breakfast dish. Serve this colorful hash on its own or topped with a fried or poached egg.

2 cups peeled and diced sweet potatoes
3 tablespoons olive oil, divided
½ teaspoon salt
4 slices thick-cut bacon, diced
1 large red bell pepper, chopped
4 sliced scallions (green parts only)
2 teaspoons smoked paprika
2 tablespoons chopped fresh parsley

1. Preheat the oven to 400°F.

2. On a large baking sheet, toss the sweet potatoes with 2 tablespoons of the olive oil and sprinkle with the salt. Roast in the preheated oven until tender, about 15 minutes.

3. While the potatoes are roasting, heat the remaining tablespoon of olive oil in a large skillet over medium-high heat. Add the bacon and reduce the heat to medium. Cook until the bacon begins to crisp, for 6 to 8 minutes. Add the bell pepper, scallions, and paprika. Cook for about 4 minutes, until the vegetables begin to soften.

4. Once the sweet potatoes are finished roasting, add them to the skillet and cook until they begin to brown, for about 8 minutes. Serve hot, garnished with parsley.

Sausage-Stuffed Kabocha Squash

SERVES 4

PREP TIME: 10 MINUTES

COOK TIME: 1 HOUR

Substitution Tip: For a dairy-free version, simply omit the cheese. If desired, sprinkle with a bit of nutritional yeast just before serving.

PER SERVING

Calories: 577
Protein: 23g
Total Fat: 33g
Saturated Fat: 9g
Carbohydrates: 52g
Fiber: 7g
Sodium: 862mg

Kabocha squash make edible cooking and serving vessels that are at once attractive and delicious. Here they're stuffed with spiced break-fast sausage mixed with fresh herbs and dried cranberries. When choosing sausage, be sure to check the ingredients and avoid those that contain gluten or are high in FODMAPs.

2 small kabocha squash, halved and seeded
3 tablespoons olive oil, divided
1¼ teaspoons salt, divided
1 teaspoon freshly ground black pepper, divided
½ pound onion- and garlic-free pork sausage
¼ cup celery, finely diced
¼ teaspoon red pepper flakes
2 tablespoons Garlic Oil (page 202)
1 tablespoon chopped fresh thyme
1 tablespoon chopped fresh rosemary
2 cups cooked quinoa
¼ cup dried cranberries
¼ cup Parmesan cheese

1. Preheat the oven to 400°F.

2. Arrange the squash halves cut-side up on a large baking sheet, drizzle them with 2 tablespoons of the olive oil, and season with ½ teaspoon each of the salt and pepper. Roast in the preheated oven for about 45 minutes, until tender.

3. Meanwhile, heat the remaining tablespoon of olive oil in a large skillet. Add the sausage and cook, breaking up with a spatula, for about 5 minutes, until browned. Add the celery, red pepper flakes, and the remainder of the salt and pepper. Cook for about 4 minutes more, until the vegetables are tender.

4. Stir in the Garlic Oil, thyme, and rosemary, then remove the skillet from the heat. Add the quinoa and cranberries, and stir to mix well.

5. Spoon the sausage mixture into the roasted squash halves and sprinkle with the cheese. Bake in the preheated oven for 10 minutes, until the cheese is melted and the filling is heated through. Serve immediately.

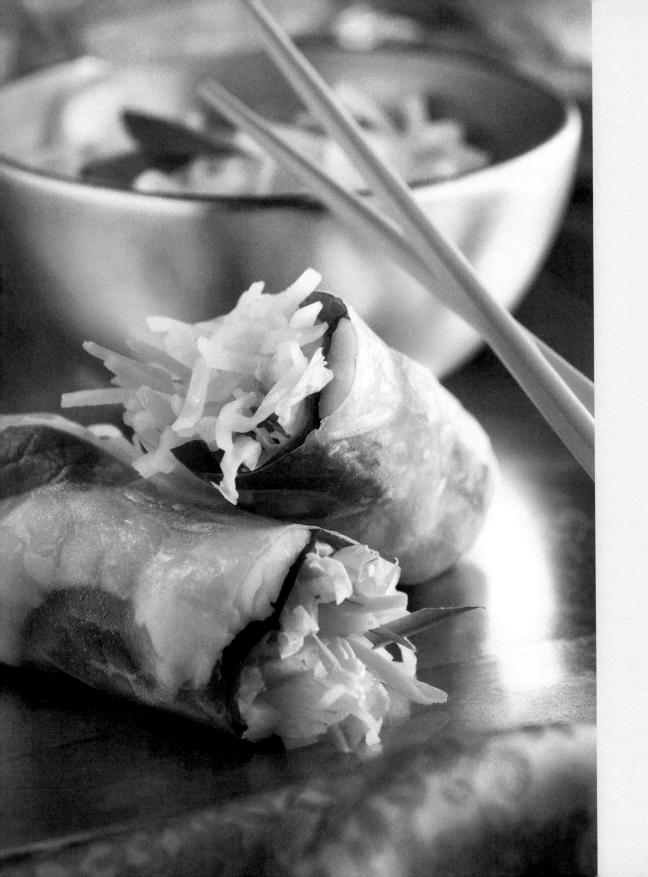

5

Snacks and Appetizers

Maple-Spiced Walnuts

MAKES ABOUT 2 CUPS

PREP TIME: 5 MINUTES

COOK TIME: 8 MINUTES

Substitution Tip: For a nut-free version, substitute pumpkin seeds for the walnuts.

PER SERVING

(¼ CUP)

Calories: 223
Protein: 8g
Total Fat: 20g
Saturated Fat: 1g
Carbohydrates: 8g
Fiber: 2g
Sodium: 242mg

These sweet, spicy nuts make a great snack on their own, but they're also a treat sprinkled over a salad or as an accompaniment to a cheese plate. They make a welcome holiday or hostess gift as well, so make a double batch if you're feeling generous.

2 tablespoons maple syrup
2 teaspoons olive oil
1 tablespoon water
2 cups walnut halves
1 tablespoon sugar
1 teaspoon coarse salt
1 teaspoon ground cumin
½ teaspoon ground coriander
⅛ teaspoon cayenne pepper

1. Combine the maple syrup, oil, and water in a large skillet. Heat, stirring, over medium heat for about 5 minutes. Stir in the walnuts.

2. Add the sugar, salt, cumin, coriander, and cayenne pepper. Cook, tossing to coat the nuts well, for about 3 minutes more, until the nuts are lightly browned.

3. Transfer to a sheet of parchment paper, spread the nuts out into a single layer, separate them, and cool completely. Serve at room temperature.

Olive Tapenade

MAKES ABOUT ¾ CUP

PREP TIME: 5 MINUTES

COOK TIME: NONE

PER SERVING

(2 TABLESPOONS)

Calories: 57
Protein: 1g
Total Fat: 5g
Saturated Fat: 1g
Carbohydrates: 4g
Fiber: 2g
Sodium: 523mg

Olives have a deep, rich umami flavor—especially helpful in seasoning when you can't use onions and garlic in your cooking. This flavorful paste is fantastic spread on gluten-free crackers or cucumber rounds. Dollop it in stew or soup to increase depth of flavor. You won't taste any fishiness from the anchovies here, but feel free to omit them if you are vegetarian or they are simply not your cup of tea.

1 cup pitted, cured black or green olives

¼ cup chopped flat-leaf parsley

1 tablespoon chopped fresh oregano

1 tablespoon capers, drained

½ teaspoon Dijon mustard

1 to 3 anchovy fillets (optional)

1 tablespoon lemon juice

1½ teaspoons Garlic Oil (page 202)

1½ teaspoons olive oil

In a blender or food processor, combine all of the ingredients and pulse to a chunky paste. You can also use a mortar and pestle to achieve the desired consistency. Serve immediately or refrigerate for up to a week.

Herbed Polenta "Fries"

MAKES 16 FRIES

PREP TIME: 5 MINUTES,
PLUS 45 MINUTES TO CHILL

COOK TIME: 40 MINUTES

Ingredient Tip: Regular
ground polenta (not
quick cooking) works best
for this recipe, but if you
are in a hurry, start with
the precooked tube, cut
it into sticks, brush the
sticks with oil, and roll in
the herbs and cheese
before broiling.

PER SERVING (4 FRIES)

Calories: 314
Protein: 14g
Total Fat: 16g
Saturated Fat: 10g
Carbohydrates: 31g
Fiber: 1g
Sodium: 656mg

Healthier than standard French fries but no less tempting, these baked cornmeal sticks can be eaten plain or dipped into Olive Tapenade (page 85) or spicy tomato sauce. They're perfect for a snack, appetizer, or side dish.

Olive oil for brushing
3¼ cups cold water
1 cup polenta
1 teaspoon chopped fresh sage
1 teaspoon chopped fresh rosemary
¾ teaspoon salt
½ cup grated Parmesan
2 tablespoons unsalted butter, cut into chunks

1. Brush an 8-by-8-inch baking dish with olive oil.

2. In a medium saucepan set over medium heat, whisk together the water, polenta, sage, rosemary, and salt and bring to a boil. Reduce the heat to medium-low and cook, stirring continuously, until the mixture thickens, for 15 to 20 minutes. Add the cheese and butter, and stir to incorporate.

3. Spoon the polenta mixture into the prepared baking dish and spread it into a flat, even layer. Refrigerate, uncovered, for about 45 minutes, until set.

4. Preheat the broiler to high and line a large baking sheet with oiled aluminum foil.

5. Invert the pan of polenta to unmold it, then cut the polenta into sticks about 4 inches by 1 inch by 1 inch. Brush the sticks with oil and arrange them in a single layer on the prepared baking sheet. Broil for 15 to 20 minutes, until golden brown and crisp. Serve immediately.

Baked Veggie Chips

SERVES 6

PREP TIME: 15 MINUTES, PLUS 15 MINUTES TO DRAIN VEGETABLES

COOK TIME: 20 MINUTES

Substitution Tip: Sweet potatoes make great chips, too. Prep and cook them the same way as the other veggies, but be sure to limit portions since sweet potatoes contain moderate levels of FODMAPs.

PER SERVING

Calories: 86
Protein: 2g
Total Fat: 1g
Saturated Fat: 0g
Carbohydrates: 20g
Fiber: 6g
Sodium: 417mg

These crispy veggie chips easily satisfy your junk-food cravings but without the subsequent guilt. Baked instead of fried and made with healthy veggies—parsnips, zucchini, and carrots—they deliver all the salty, crunchy satisfaction of a bag of chips.

2 medium parsnips, peeled
2 medium zucchini
2 medium carrots, peeled
Olive oil spray
1 teaspoon salt, plus more for garnish

1. Using a handheld mandoline or a very sharp knife, slice the vegetables into very thin (1/16-inch) rounds.

2. Preheat the oven to 375°F.

3. Lightly oil 2 large baking sheets with olive oil spray.

4. Arrange the sliced vegetables on paper towels in a single layer, season with 1 teaspoon of salt, and let sit for 15 minutes. Dry the vegetables as thoroughly as possible with a paper towel.

5. Arrange the vegetable slices on the baking sheets in a single layer and coat with additional olive oil spray. Bake in the preheated oven for about 20 minutes.

6. Remove the chips from the oven, sprinkle them with additional salt, and let cool for 5 minutes. Serve immediately or cool to room temperature. The chips can then be stored in a sealed container on the countertop for up to 3 days.

Spiced Tortilla Chips

SERVES 4 TO 6

PREP TIME: 10 MINUTES

COOK TIME: 15 MINUTES

Substitution Tip: For a different flavor, leave out the cumin and chili powder, and replace the plain vegetable oil with Garlic Oil (page 202), or simply omit the spices and season with salt.

PER SERVING

Calories: 189
Protein: 4g
Total Fat: 6g
Saturated Fat: 1g
Carbohydrates: 32g
Fiber: 5g
Sodium: 615mg

These crispy, lightly spiced tortilla chips make a perfect snack on their own but also a great vehicle for any salsa or dip in this chapter, particularly the Pineapple Salsa (page 97) and Spiced Carrot Dip (page 96).

12 (6-inch) corn tortillas
1 tablespoon vegetable oil
1 teaspoon ground cumin
1 teaspoon gluten-free, onion- and garlic-free chili powder
1 teaspoon salt

1. Preheat the oven to 350°F.

2. Cut each tortilla into 8 wedges. Brush the wedges on both sides with the oil and arrange them in a single layer on a large baking sheet.

3. In a small dish, combine the cumin, chili powder, and salt. Sprinkle the spice mixture onto the chips, distributing evenly.

4. Bake the chips for about 7 minutes. Turn the pan around and bake for an additional 7 to 8 minutes, until the chips are golden brown and crisp. Serve immediately or cool to room temperature. Cooled chips may be stored in a sealed container on the countertop for up to 3 days.

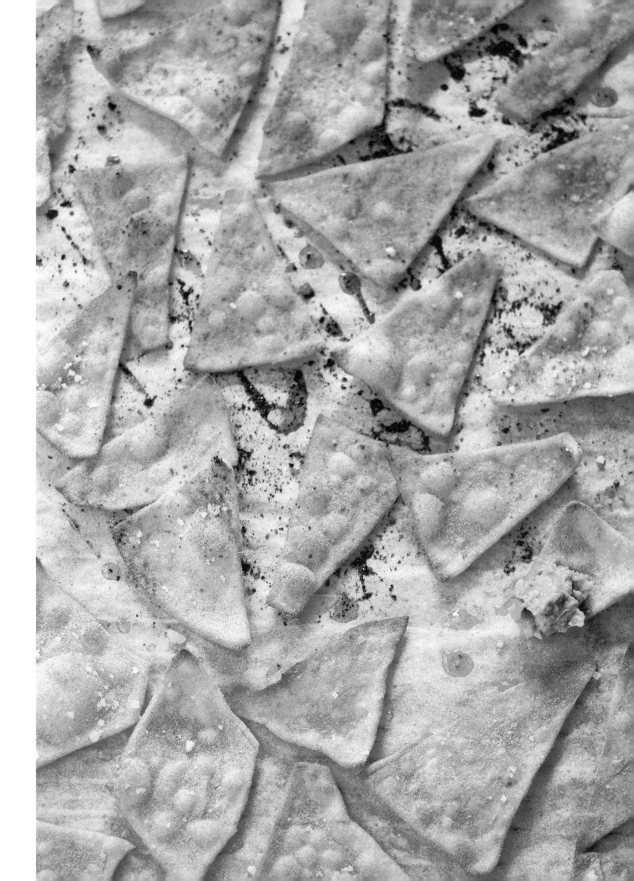

Smoked Trout Brandade

SERVES 6 TO 8

PREP TIME: 10 MINUTES

COOK TIME: 35 MINUTES

Substitution Tip: For a dairy-free version, substitute rice milk for the lactose-free milk and omit the Parmesan cheese.

PER SERVING

Calories: 239
Protein: 14g
Total Fat: 14g
Saturated Fat: 3g
Carbohydrates: 15g
Fiber: 2g
Sodium: 290mg

Traditional brandade is an emulsion of potatoes, olive oil, and salted cod, which needs to be soaked for a long period of time. Using smoked trout instead of cod cuts the soaking out of the equation, making this a much quicker dish to prepare, plus the smokiness of the fish brings an additional layer of flavor to the salty, garlicky spread—a tasty bonus. Serve it spread on toasted rounds of gluten-free baguette with fresh or oven-roasted tomatoes.

1 pound russet potatoes, peeled and cut into chunks
8 ounces smoked trout, skin and bones removed, flaked into small pieces
¾ cup lactose-free milk
2 tablespoons lemon juice
¼ cup olive oil
2 tablespoons Garlic Oil (page 202)
½ teaspoon salt
½ teaspoon freshly ground black pepper
2 tablespoons freshly grated Parmesan cheese

1. Bring a large saucepan of water to a boil over high heat. Add the potatoes and cook for 15 to 20 minutes, until they are tender. Drain potatoes and set aside.

2. Preheat the oven to 400°F.

3. In a large bowl, combine the trout and milk, and mash to a paste. Add the lemon juice and the cooked potatoes, and stir with a fork until well combined. Add the olive oil, Garlic Oil, salt, and pepper, and mix thoroughly. Taste and adjust the seasoning as needed.

4. Spoon the mixture into a shallow baking dish, top with the cheese, and bake in the preheated oven for about 15 minutes, until the cheese is melted and golden brown. Serve hot.

Herbed Veggie-and-Tofu Skewers

MAKES 10 TO 12 SKEWERS

PREP TIME: 15 MINUTES,
PLUS 15 MINUTES TO DRAIN
THE TOFU AND OVERNIGHT
TO MARINATE

COOK TIME: 10 MINUTES

Substitution Tip: To make
a soy-free version, omit
the tofu and substitute
cubes of blanched
potatoes marinated in
the vinegar-mustard
mixture.

PER SERVING (2 SKEWERS)

Calories: 274
Protein: 18g
Total Fat: 18g
Saturated Fat: 2g
Carbohydrates: 14g
Fiber: 6g
Sodium: 474mg

Freezing and then thawing tofu changes its texture, creating small pockets that cause it to act like a sponge and soak up marinades and sauces. Here the frozen and thawed tofu is marinated overnight in a mixture of fresh herbs, balsamic vinegar, and Dijon mustard. It's then grilled along with fresh vegetables for a healthy vegetarian barbecue appetizer or main dish.

28 ounces extra-firm tofu, drained, frozen, and thawed
¼ cup balsamic vinegar
1 tablespoon Dijon mustard
1½ teaspoons chopped fresh thyme
3 tablespoons olive oil, plus more for oiling
1 teaspoon Garlic Oil (page 202)
1 tablespoon lemon juice
1 teaspoon coarse salt
Pinch cayenne pepper
1 globe eggplant (about 1 pound), cut into ½-inch chunks
1 green bell pepper, cut into 1-inch squares
1 red bell pepper, cut into 1-inch squares

1. Cut the block of tofu into 4 or 5 slabs, and place them on a towel-lined baking sheet. Place another towel and then another baking sheet on top, and weight it with several cans of tomatoes or other heavy items. Let sit for 15 to 20 minutes to drain excess water.

2. Cut the drained tofu into 1-inch cubes.

3. In a large bowl, combine the vinegar, mustard, and thyme, and stir to mix well. Add the cubed tofu and toss gently to coat well. Cover and refrigerate overnight.

4. Heat a grill or grill pan to medium-high heat. ▶

5. In a large bowl, stir together the olive oil, Garlic Oil, lemon juice, salt, and cayenne. Add the eggplant and bell peppers, and toss to coat.

6. Thread the tofu cubes and vegetable chunks onto skewers, alternating and distributing the ingredients evenly.

7. Grill the skewers, turning every few minutes, until the tofu is browned and the veggies are tender, for 8 to 10 minutes total. Serve immediately.

Herbed Rice Fritters with Parmesan Cheese

SERVES 4

PREP TIME: 10 MINUTES,
PLUS 30 MINUTES TO
CHILL CAKES

COOK TIME: 16 MINUTES

Substitution Tip: For a dairy-free, egg-free version, omit the cheese and replace the egg with a chia-seed egg replacer: Grind 1 tablespoon white chia-seed meal in a food processor or spice grinder, and mix with 3 tablespoons warm water. Let the mixture stand for 5 to 10 minutes, until it thickens and becomes the consistency of raw eggs.

PER SERVING

Calories: 458
Protein: 15g
Total Fat: 22g
Saturated Fat: 7g
Carbohydrates: 53g
Fiber: 3g
Sodium: 574mg

These crispy fritters are similar to Italian arancini, *which are made with leftover risotto. This version uses cooked brown rice, but if you have leftover risotto, by all means, feel free to use it instead. Be sure to use a gluten-free flour blend that is made with only low-FODMAP grains and starches, such as King Arthur's.*

2 cups cooked brown rice
½ cup freshly grated Parmesan cheese
1 tablespoon chopped fresh oregano
½ teaspoon salt
¼ teaspoon freshly ground black pepper
1 egg, lightly beaten
½ cup gluten-free all-purpose flour
¼ cup olive oil
Finely chopped fresh parsley

1. In a medium bowl, stir together the rice, Parmesan cheese, oregano, salt, pepper, and egg.

2. With slightly wet hands, form the mixture into eight cakes, about 2 inches in diameter. Place the cakes on a plate, cover with plastic wrap, and refrigerate for 30 minutes.

3. Place the flour on a plate and coat the chilled cakes in it.

4. Heat the olive oil in a large skillet over medium-high heat and cook the cakes, 4 at a time, until golden brown, for about 4 minutes per side. Garnish with the parsley and serve immediately.

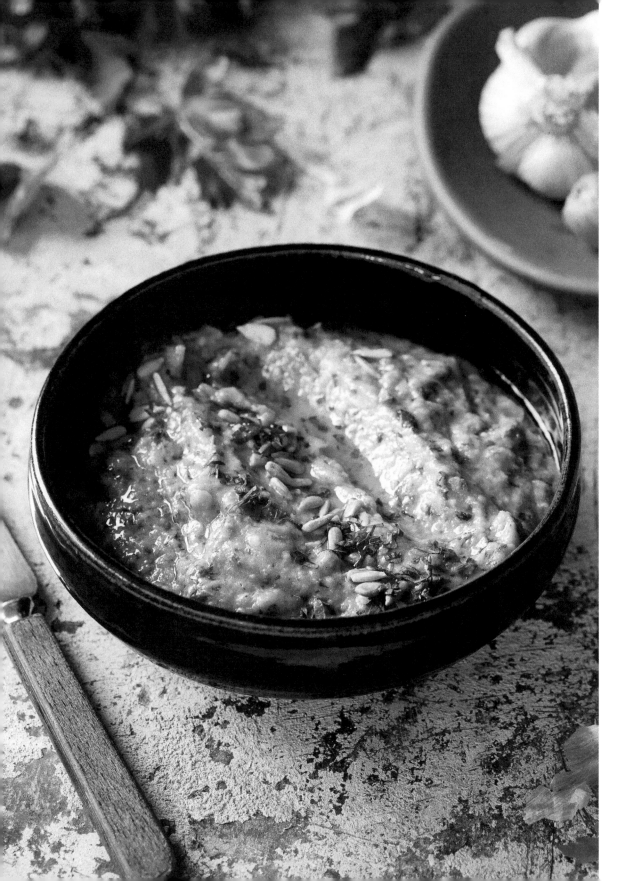

Smoky Eggplant Dip

MAKES ABOUT 2 CUPS

PREP TIME: 10 MINUTES

COOK TIME: 20 MINUTES

Substitution Tip: If you are allergic to nuts, simply omit the peanut butter or substitute sunflower-seed butter.

PER SERVING

(½ CUP)

Calories: 105
Protein: 4g
Total Fat: 5g
Saturated Fat: 1g
Carbohydrates: 11g
Fiber: 6g
Sodium: 200mg

This smoky dip or spread is similar to Middle Eastern baba ghanoush but replaces high-FODMAP tahini and garlic with peanut butter and Garlic Oil (page 202). Serve it with gluten-free bread or crudités for dipping, or spread it on a wrap with roasted veggies.

1 large eggplant (about 1 pound)
¼ cup finely chopped fresh flat-leaf parsley, plus more for garnish
2 tablespoons creamy peanut butter
2 tablespoons lemon juice
¼ teaspoon salt
2 to 4 tablespoons Garlic Oil (page 202)
1 tablespoon minced fresh parsley
1 tablespoon toasted sunflower seeds

1. Preheat the oven to 450°F.

2. Line a large baking sheet with aluminum foil. Prick the eggplant all over with the tines of a fork and place it on the prepared baking sheet. Bake in the preheated oven for about 20 minutes, until the skin begins to brown and blister and the flesh inside is soft. Remove from the oven and let sit until cool enough to handle. Halve the eggplant lengthwise and scoop out the flesh, discarding the skin.

3. In a food processor, combine the eggplant flesh, parsley, peanut butter, lemon juice, and salt, and process until smooth. With the processor running, add 2 tablespoons of the Garlic Oil. Add additional oil, if needed, to achieve the desired consistency. Spoon into a serving dish, garnish with parsley, sunflower seeds, and additional Garlic Oil, and serve immediately.

Spiced Carrot Dip

SERVES 6 TO 8

PREP TIME: 10 MINUTES

COOK TIME: 20 MINUTES

Substitution Tip: For a vegan or dairy-free version, omit the feta cheese.

PER SERVING

Calories: 175
Protein: 3g
Total Fat: 11g
Saturated Fat: 3g
Carbohydrates: 17g
Fiber: 4g
Sodium: 459mg

A handful of pantry staples can be quickly transformed into this delicious and stunningly bright appetizer. Serve this dip with gluten-free crackers or baguette rounds, or with crudités for dipping. Or include in a meze platter.

2 pounds carrots, peeled and cut into 3-inch lengths
¼ cup olive oil
¼ cup red-wine vinegar
2 tablespoons Garlic Oil (page 202)
1 teaspoon onion- and garlic-free chili paste
1 teaspoon ground cumin
½ teaspoon ground ginger
½ teaspoon salt
2 ounces feta cheese, crumbled
6 pitted black olives, chopped

1. Fill a large saucepan halfway with salted water and bring to a boil over high heat. Reduce the heat to medium, add the carrots, and cook for 15 to 20 minutes, until the carrots are tender.

2. In a food processor, process the carrots, olive oil, vinegar, Garlic Oil, chili paste, cumin, ginger, and salt to a smooth purée.

3. Spoon the purée into a serving dish, top with the crumbled feta cheese and olives, and serve immediately.

Pineapple Salsa

MAKES ABOUT 2 CUPS

PREP TIME: 5 MINUTES,
PLUS 20 MINUTES TO REST

COOK TIME: NONE

Ingredient Tip: Fresh pineapple is your best choice here, but canned pineapple in its own juice is a fine substitute when the fresh fruit is unavailable. You can also substitute other fruits, such as melon, or use a combination.

PER SERVING

(½ CUP)

Calories: 73
Protein: 1g
Total Fat: 4g
Saturated Fat: 1g
Carbohydrates: 11g
Fiber: 1g
Sodium: 292mg

This fruity, tropical salsa offers a delightful balance of sweet and spice. Serve it with Spiced Tortilla Chips (page 88) or use it for topping tacos. It also makes a great sauce for grilled or roasted fish or chicken.

2 cups chopped pineapple
2 jalapeño chiles, seeded and finely chopped
¼ cup finely chopped cilantro
½ teaspoon salt
Juice of 1 lime
1 tablespoon olive oil

In a medium bowl, stir all of the ingredients together until well combined. Let sit at room temperature for 15 to 20 minutes before serving to allow the flavors to blend.

Vietnamese Shrimp-and-Herb Spring Rolls

SERVES 4

PREP TIME: 5 MINUTES,
PLUS 1 HOUR
MARINATING TIME

COOK TIME: 50 MINUTES

Substitution Tip: For a shellfish-free version, replace the shrimp with cooked chicken, fish, tofu, or additional vegetables. Grilled or roasted eggplant, zucchini, and bell peppers would all be good choices.

PER SERVING

Calories: 450
Protein: 25g
Total Fat: 4g
Saturated Fat: 0g
Carbohydrates: 62g
Fiber: 4g
Sodium: 1577mg

These fresh, flavorful spring rolls make a great snack, appetizer, or even a light entrée. Be creative with the filling, substituting any meat, fish, or vegetable for the shrimp. You can adjust the flavor by adding other herbs, such as fresh basil, or if you like, add crushed peanuts for some crunch or thinly sliced fresh chiles for a bit of a kick.

FOR THE DIPPING SAUCE
¼ cup rice vinegar
¼ cup fish sauce
1 cup water
1 tablespoon sugar

FOR THE SPRING ROLLS
16 round rice-paper wrappers
1 cup fresh mint leaves
8 ounces cooked shrimp, peeled and halved lengthwise
2 cups cooked and cooled thin rice noodles
16 small lettuce leaves
3 cups bean sprouts
1 cup cilantro leaves

1. To make the sauce, combine the vinegar, fish sauce, water, and sugar in a small saucepan set over medium heat. Cook, stirring, until the sugar is fully dissolved, for about 5 minutes. Remove from the heat and let cool completely.

2. Fill a wide, shallow bowl with warm water. Dunk 2 rice papers at a time into the water and let sit for about 1 minute, until softened. Lift the rice papers out of the water carefully and lay them, one on top of the other, on a clean dish towel.

3. Lay about 4 mint leaves in a line at the bottom of the rice paper, then add 4 shrimp halves on top of the mint. Top with a small handful of the rice noodles, a lettuce leaf, a small handful of bean sprouts, and a few cilantro leaves.

4. Fold the sides over the filling, then roll the rice paper up like a burrito and set on a serving platter, seam-side down.

5. Repeat with the remaining ingredients until you have 8 rolls. Halve the rolls and serve immediately, along with the dipping sauce.

Spicy Chicken Wings

SERVES 8 TO 10

PREP TIME: 5 MINUTES,
PLUS 1 HOUR
MARINATING TIME

COOK TIME: 50 MINUTES

Ingredient Tip: When
buying hot-pepper sauce,
check the ingredients to
be sure it is free of
FODMAPs. Many hot
sauces contain garlic or
garlic powder, both of
which are off limits.
Tabasco, Crystal, Texas
Pete's, and Trappey's
Red Devil are all suitable.

PER SERVING

Calories: 741
Protein: 82g
Total Fat: 42g
Saturated Fat: 7g
Carbohydrates: 4g
Fiber: 0g
Sodium: 244mg

Nothing beats spicy chicken wings as a game-day—or any-day—snack. Most wing recipes include high-FODMAP garlic or garlic powder, but this one has neither. Make a big batch the next time you invite the gang over to watch the big game or whenever you're looking for an easy and satisfying snack for a crowd.

⅔ cup hot-pepper sauce (see Ingredient Tip)
⅔ cup canola oil or nondairy butter substitute
1 teaspoon cayenne pepper
3 tablespoons rice vinegar or white wine vinegar
5 pounds chicken wings, separated at the joint and
  with the tip snipped off

1. To make the sauce, combine the hot-pepper sauce, oil, cayenne, and vinegar in a small saucepan, and cook over low heat until the mixture begins to boil. Remove from the heat and let cool.

2. In a large bowl, toss the wings with the sauce until well coated. Cover and refrigerate for 1 hour.

3. Preheat the oven to 400°F.

4. Drain the wings, reserving the marinade, and arrange them in a single layer on a large baking sheet. Bake in the preheated oven for 30 minutes. Turn the wings over and bake for 20 minutes more, until they begin to brown.

5. While the wings are in the oven, heat the reserved marinade in a saucepan over high heat and bring to a boil. Simmer for 15 minutes.

6. Serve the wings hot with extra sauce for dipping.

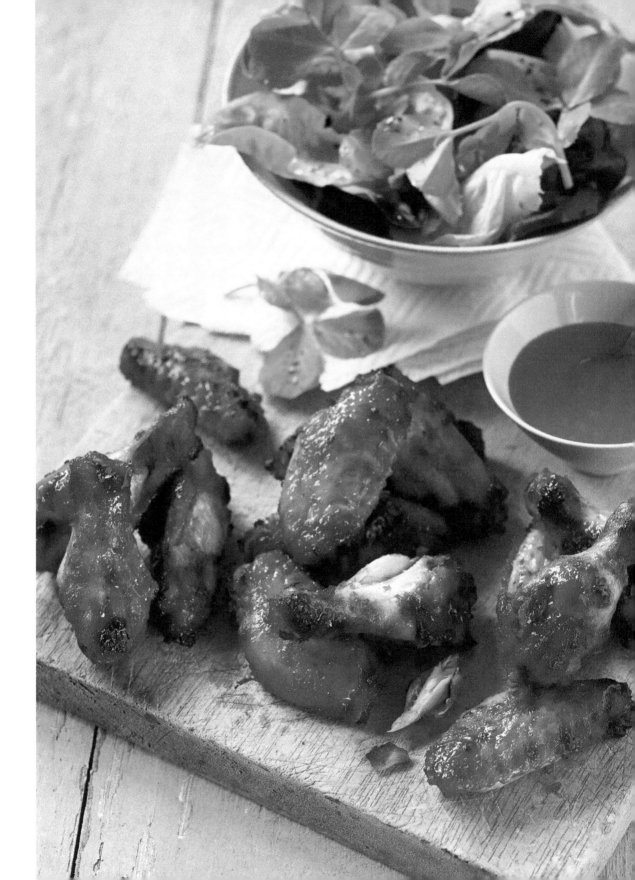

Chinese Chicken in Lettuce Cups

SERVES 4

PREP TIME: 10 MINUTES

COOK TIME: 5 MINUTES

Substitution Tip: For a soy-free version, replace the soy sauce with coconut aminos.

PER SERVING

Calories: 378
Protein: 36g
Total Fat: 19g
Saturated Fat: 4g
Carbohydrates: 14g
Fiber: 1g
Sodium: 778mg

Minced chicken cooked with ginger and water chestnuts makes a flavorful filling for crisp lettuce cups. Serve this as a passed appetizer (using small lettuce leaves) or a first course. As an alternative to minced chicken, you can substitute just about any ground meat, such as turkey, pork, beef, or lamb.

2 tablespoons gluten-free soy sauce
2 tablespoons rice vinegar
½ teaspoon salt
½ teaspoon sugar
2 tablespoons vegetable oil
2 teaspoons Garlic Oil (page 202)
2 teaspoons minced fresh ginger
1 pound boneless, skinless chicken breasts, minced
½ cup water chestnuts, minced
8 to 10 inner leaves iceberg lettuce, edges trimmed and chilled
Handful of fresh cilantro leaves, coarsely chopped
¼ cup unsalted roasted peanuts, coarsely chopped (optional)

1. In a small bowl, stir together the soy sauce, rice vinegar, salt, and sugar.

2. Heat the vegetable oil and Garlic Oil in a skillet or wok set over high heat. Add the ginger and cook, stirring, for 10 seconds. Add the chicken and cook, stirring, for about 1 minute, until the chicken is opaque all over. Add the water chestnuts and reduce to medium-low. Stir in the soy sauce mixture and cook for about 2 minutes more, until the chicken is cooked through.

3. Arrange the lettuce cups on a platter or serving plates and spoon some of the chicken mixture into each, dividing equally. Garnish each serving with cilantro and peanuts, if using, and serve immediately.

Lamb Meatballs

PREP TIME: 15 MINUTES

COOK TIME: 20 MINUTES

Substitution Tip: For a dairy-free, egg-free version, omit the cheese and replace the egg with a chia-seed egg replacer: Grind 1 tablespoon white chia-seed meal in a food processor or spice grinder and mix with 3 tablespoons warm water. Let the mixture stand for 5 to 10 minutes, until it thickens and becomes the consistency of raw eggs.

PER SERVING

Calories: 361
Protein: 37g
Total Fat: 13g
Saturated Fat: 6g
Carbohydrates: 21g
Fiber: 1g
Sodium: 844mg

These meatballs make a great appetizer, or try them with a fresh tomato sauce on top of gluten-free pasta. They also work as an excellent sandwich filling on a gluten-free roll. You can make the balls bigger or smaller depending on how you intend to serve them, but keep in mind that different sizes may require you to adjust cooking times.

Oil for preparing the pan
1 pound ground lamb
½ cup cooked rice
⅓ cup crumbled feta cheese
Zest of 1 lemon
3 tablespoons minced parsley
1 teaspoon salt
1 teaspoon ground cumin
1 teaspoon ground allspice
½ teaspoon ground cinnamon
1 egg, lightly beaten
1 tablespoon Garlic Oil (page 202)

1. Preheat the oven to 400°F.

2. Line a large, rimmed baking sheet with lightly oiled parchment paper.

3. In a mixing bowl, combine the lamb, rice, cheese, lemon zest, parsley, salt, cumin, allspice, cinnamon, and egg, and mix well.

4. Form the lamb mixture into 1½-inch balls and arrange them on the prepared baking sheet.

5. Bake the meatballs in the preheated oven until they are browned and cooked through, for about 20 minutes.

6. Drizzle the Garlic Oil over the meatballs just before serving and serve hot.

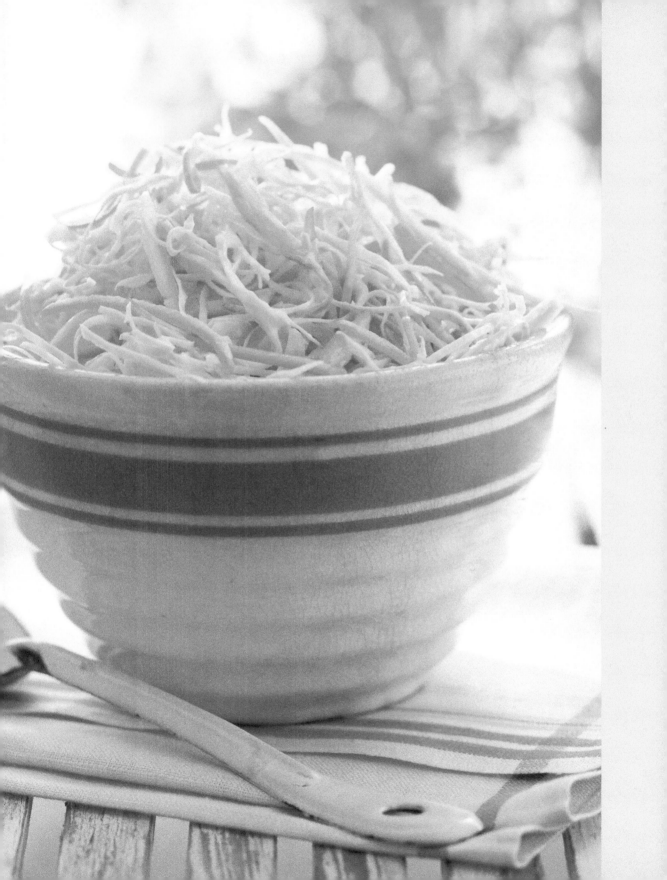

6
Side Dishes

Classic Coleslaw

SERVES 6 TO 8

PREP TIME: 10 MINUTES,
PLUS 2 HOURS TO CHILL

COOK TIME: NONE

Substitution Tip: If you
follow a soy-free diet, be
sure to use a soy-free
mayonnaise or make your
own Homemade Mayon-
naise (page 204).

PER SERVING

Calories: 198
Protein: 5g
Total Fat: 14g
Saturated Fat: 2g
Carbohydrates: 19g
Fiber: 4g
Sodium: 694mg

Crisp, vinegary, and a little sweet and spicy, this coleslaw provides the perfect side dish for barbecued or grilled meats, fish, or seafood. It also makes a great picnic dish and a refreshing accompaniment to hot dogs, burgers, or sandwiches.

1 cup mayonnaise
3 tablespoons Dijon mustard
1 tablespoon white-wine vinegar
Juice of 1 lemon
Pinch sugar
½ teaspoon celery seed
Several dashes onion- and garlic-free hot-pepper sauce
¾ teaspoon salt
½ teaspoon freshly ground black pepper
1 head green cabbage, shredded
2 carrots, grated
1 fresh red chile, sliced

In a large bowl, combine the mayonnaise, mustard, vinegar, lemon juice, sugar, celery seed, hot sauce, salt, and pepper, and stir together. Add the cabbage and carrots to the dressing, and toss together until evenly coated. Cover and chill the coleslaw for at least 2 hours before serving.

Seared Green Beans with Sesame Oil

SERVES 4

PREP TIME: 5 MINUTES

COOK TIME: 10 MINUTES

Ingredient Tip: When buying sesame oil, be sure you are buying 100 percent pure sesame oil rather than vegetable oil merely flavored with sesame oil. For optimal flavor, purchase the best brand available—a little sesame oil goes a long way, so spending a little extra will be worth it. Dark sesame oil is specified for this recipe; it has a deep, nutty flavor.

PER SERVING

Calories: 113
Protein: 3g
Total Fat: 7g
Saturated Fat: 1g
Carbohydrates: 12g
Fiber: 6g
Sodium: 49mg

Just three ingredients are all you need to make this addictive side dish. First you blanch the green beans in boiling water to make them tender, then quickly sear them in hot sesame oil, for an infusion of nutty, smoky flavor. Serve them with Asian-style fish or poultry dishes.

1½ pounds green beans, trimmed
2 tablespoons dark sesame oil
Salt

1. Bring a large saucepan of salted water to a boil over high heat. Add the green beans and cook just until tender but still bright green, for 2 to 3 minutes. Drain well.

2. Heat the oil in a large skillet over high heat. When the oil is very hot, add the green beans (you might have to cook the beans in batches to avoid crowding the pan), tossing occasionally, for 3 to 4 minutes, until the beans begin to blacken and blister in spots. Transfer to a serving platter and sprinkle with salt. Serve hot.

Lemony Grilled Zucchini with Feta and Pine Nuts

SERVES 4

PREP TIME: 5 MINUTES

COOK TIME: 8 MINUTES

Substitution Tip: For a dairy-free version, replace the feta cheese with chopped, pitted olives. For a nut-free version, omit the pine nuts.

PER SERVING

Calories: 176
Protein: 3g
Total Fat: 15g
Saturated Fat: 5g
Carbohydrates: 7g
Fiber: 2g
Sodium: 836mg

Grilling zucchini gives it a touch of smoky flavor and a luscious texture. Spiked with a lemon dressing and tangy crumbled feta cheese, this refreshing side dish is a perfect accompaniment to grilled or roasted meats or fish. For added color, substitute some of the zucchini with other summer squashes, like yellow squash or pattypan squash.

3 ounces feta, crumbled
2 tablespoons chopped fresh mint leaves
2 tablespoons olive oil, divided
1 teaspoon fresh lemon juice
1 teaspoon lemon zest
2 scallions, green parts only, thinly sliced
2-3 zucchini (about 1½ pounds), halved lengthwise and cut into 3-inch pieces
1 teaspoon salt
2 tablespoons toasted pine nuts

1. In a small bowl, stir together the feta, mint, 1 tablespoon of the oil, lemon juice, lemon zest, and scallions.

2. Brush the remaining tablespoon of oil onto the zucchini and sprinkle with the salt.

3. Heat a grill or grill pan to high heat. Cook the zucchini for 3 to 4 minutes per side, until grill marks appear and the zucchini is tender. Transfer the cooked zucchini to a serving platter, and spoon the topping over the top. Sprinkle the pine nuts over the top and serve immediately.

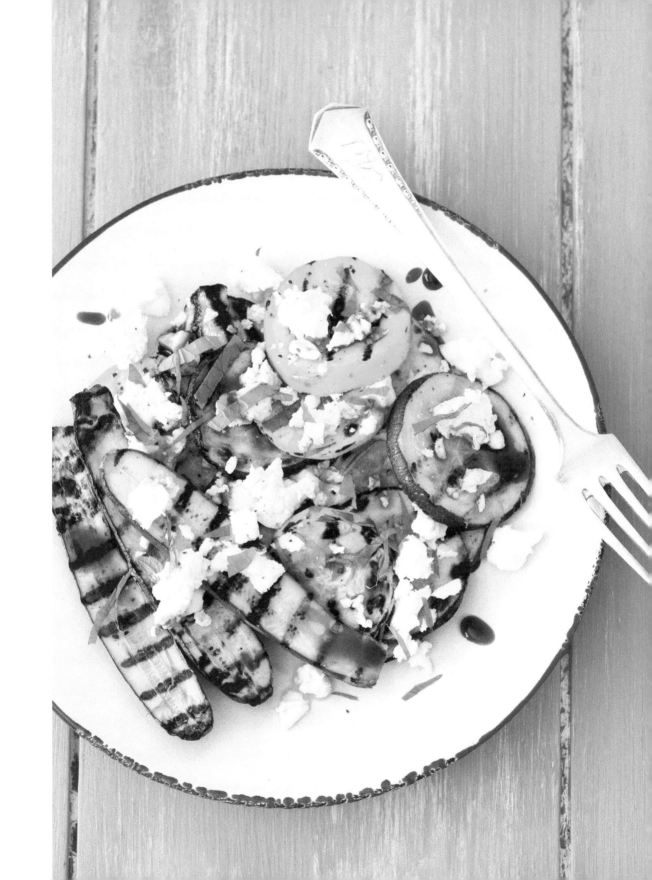

Caramelized Fennel

SERVES 4

PREP TIME: 10 MINUTES

COOK TIME: 60 MINUTES

Substitution Tip: For a dairy-free version, simply omit the Parmesan cheese.

PER SERVING

Calories: 228
Protein: 8g
Total Fat: 16g
Saturated Fat: 4g
Carbohydrates: 18g
Fiber: 7g
Sodium: 836mg

Lovers of caramelized onions will rejoice in this side dish. Fennel has a completely different flavor than onion does, but when caramelized, it provides the same deep, rich, savory sweetness. This dish uses only the bulb of the fennel, but trim off the leafy tops, and you can use them in place of fresh dill or other herbs.

¼ cup olive oil
4 large fennel bulbs, cut into ¼-inch-thick slices
1 teaspoon salt
¼ cup freshly grated Parmesan
2 tablespoons chopped fresh parsley
1 teaspoon lemon zest
2 teaspoons lemon juice

1. In a large, heavy skillet, heat the olive oil over medium-high heat. Stir in the fennel and salt, reduce the heat to medium, and cook, stirring occasionally, for 45 to 60 minutes, lowering the heat if needed, until the fennel is golden brown and very tender.

2. Just before serving, stir in the cheese, parsley, lemon zest, and lemon juice.

Green Beans and New Potatoes with Tomato

SERVES 8

PREP TIME: 10 MINUTES

COOK TIME: 10 MINUTES

Cooking Tip: To speed your prep, just snap off the stem end of each green bean; if there's a sturdy string, it will come off right along with it.

PER SERVING

Calories: 244
Protein: 7g
Total Fat: 4g
Saturated Fat: 1g
Carbohydrates: 49g
Fiber: 11g
Sodium: 615mg

Crisp, tender green beans are a fitting complement for grilled, braised, or roasted meats. This hearty dish, with bright, fresh tomatoes and velvety chunks of potato, is all you need to round out a roasted-chicken dinner.

1 tablespoon olive oil
1 tablespoon Garlic Oil (page 202)
1¼ pounds green beans, trimmed
1½ cups diced red new potatoes
1 teaspoon salt
¼ cup water
⅓ cup chopped cilantro
¾ pound plum tomatoes, peeled and coarsely chopped
¼ teaspoon freshly ground black pepper
¼ teaspoon cayenne

1. Heat the olive oil and Garlic Oil in a large skillet over medium-high heat. Add the green beans, potatoes, and salt, and cook, stirring, for 1 minute.

2. Stir in the water, cover the pan, and cook until the beans are barely tender, about 5 minutes.

3. Stir in the cilantro and tomatoes, cover the pan again, reduce the heat to low, and cook for about 4 minutes more, until the tomatoes begin to break down.

4. Just before serving, stir in the pepper and cayenne. Serve hot.

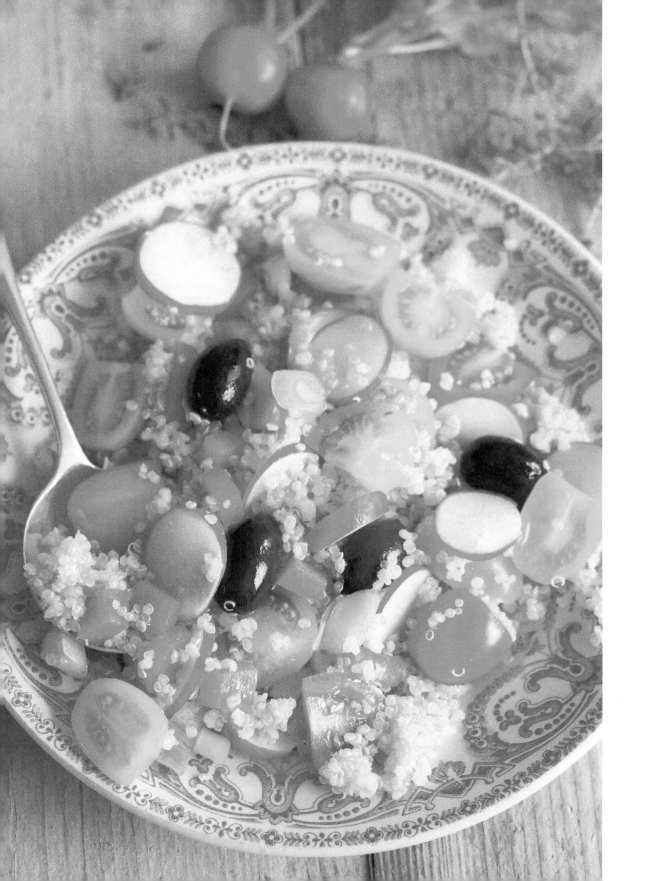

Quinoa with Cherry Tomatoes, Olives, and Radishes

SERVES 4

PREP TIME: 10 MINUTES

COOK TIME: 20 MINUTES

Ingredient Tip: You can use golden, red, or black quinoa for this dish. Check the cooking directions on the package to make sure the cooking time is the same.

PER SERVING

Calories: 309
Protein: 7g
Total Fat: 19g
Saturated Fat: 3g
Carbohydrates: 31g
Fiber: 5g
Sodium: 886mg

This simple, summery quinoa dish is easy to make and very satisfying. Feel free to add fresh herbs, such as basil or oregano, or other vegetables like cucumber, bell peppers, or thinly sliced celery.

1 cup uncooked quinoa
1 teaspoon salt
¼ cup white wine vinegar or white balsamic vinegar
¼ cup olive oil
1 cup cherry tomatoes, halved or quartered
1 cup pitted cured black olives, halved, quartered, or left whole if small
4 to 6 radishes, thinly sliced

1. In a medium saucepan, combine the quinoa and salt with 2 cups water and bring to a boil. Reduce the heat to low, cover, and let simmer for 15 to 20 minutes, until tender.

2. Meanwhile, in a small bowl, whisk together the vinegar and olive oil. When the quinoa is cooked, immediately toss it together with the dressing in a large bowl. Add the tomatoes, olives, and radishes and toss together. Serve immediately or refrigerate, covered, for up to 3 days.

Roasted Lemon-Parmesan Broccoli

SERVES 6

PREP TIME: 10 MINUTES

COOK TIME: 25 MINUTES

Substitution Tip: For a dairy-free version, omit the Parmesan cheese. Instead, substitute 2 tablespoons of nutritional yeast, if desired. For a nut-free version, omit the pine nuts.

PER SERVING

Calories: 117
Protein: 5g
Total Fat: 8g
Saturated Fat: 2g
Carbohydrates: 9g
Fiber: 3g
Sodium: 500mg

This recipe offers a simple concept for turning plain broccoli into a memorable dish. Roasting broccoli makes the edges deliciously crispy, while lemon and Parmesan balance out broccoli's bitter edge with just the right touch of salty, tangy, and sweet.

1½ pounds broccoli, cut into florets
2 tablespoons olive oil
1 teaspoon salt
½ teaspoon freshly ground black pepper
2 teaspoons grated lemon zest
2 tablespoons lemon juice
¼ cup freshly grated Parmesan cheese
2 tablespoons toasted pine nuts

1. Preheat the oven to 425°F.

2. On a large, rimmed sheet pan, toss the broccoli with the olive oil, sprinkle with salt and pepper, and spread into a single layer. Roast in the preheated oven for about 25 minutes, until the broccoli begins to brown on the edges.

3. Transfer the broccoli to a large serving platter and toss with the lemon zest, lemon juice, and cheese. Garnish with the pine nuts and serve immediately.

Rice Pilaf with Vegetables

SERVES 4

PREP TIME: 5 MINUTES, PLUS
15 MINUTES RESTING TIME

COOK TIME: 25 MINUTES

Substitution Tip: Feel free
to substitute brown rice
for the white rice. Keep in
mind that you may need
to cook the brown rice
longer.

PER SERVING

Calories: 405
Protein: 11g
Total Fat: 2g
Saturated Fat: 0g
Carbohydrates: 85g
Fiber: 3g
Sodium: 1648mg

Rice pilaf transforms boring rice into a lovely side dish. This version is flavored with Garlic Oil and saffron and studded with crisp, tender green beans, golden raisins, and red bell pepper.

1 tablespoon Garlic Oil (page 202)
½ medium red bell pepper, finely chopped
2 teaspoons salt, divided
2 cups long-grain white rice
Pinch saffron threads steeped in ¼ cup hot (not boiling) water
2½ cups homemade (onion- and garlic-free) vegetable or chicken broth
2 bay leaves
1 cup fresh or frozen green beans, cut into 2-inch pieces
¼ cup golden raisins

1. Preheat the oven to 350°F.

2. Heat the Garlic Oil in a medium, oven-safe saucepan over medium heat. Add the bell pepper and ½ teaspoon of the salt and cook, stirring, for 3 to 4 minutes, until the pepper begins to soften.

3. Add the rice and cook, stirring frequently, until the rice just begins to brown, for about 3 minutes.

4. Add the saffron threads and their soaking water, broth, bay leaves, and the remaining 1½ teaspoons salt. Increase the heat and bring to a boil.

5. Scatter the green beans over the top of the rice, cover the pan, and bake in the preheated oven for 15 minutes. Remove the pan from the oven and let rest, without removing the lid, for 15 minutes. Just before serving, fluff with a fork and stir in the raisins. Serve hot.

Coconut Rice

SERVES 4

PREP TIME: 5 MINUTES,
PLUS 10 MINUTES
RESTING TIME

COOK TIME: 30 MINUTES

Cooking Tip: Before cooking white rice, always rinse it in cold, running water until the water runs clear.

PER SERVING

Calories: 416
Protein: 7g
Total Fat: 8g
Saturated Fat: 0g
Carbohydrates: 76g
Fiber: 1g
Sodium: 610mg

This coconut-flavored rice is the perfect accompaniment to savory grilled meat dishes like chicken satay or barbecued pork. For even more coconut flavor, stir in ½ cup shredded coconut along with the coconut milk.

2 cups jasmine rice
1 cup water
1 (14-ounce) can light coconut milk
1 teaspoon salt

1. In a medium saucepan, combine the rice, water, coconut milk, and salt, and bring to a boil over high heat. Reduce the heat to low, cover, and cook for 30 to 40 minutes, until the rice is tender and the liquid has evaporated.

2. Remove the pot from the heat and let the rice rest, without taking the lid off, for about 10 minutes. Just before serving, fluff with a fork. Serve hot.

Sesame Rice Noodles

SERVES 4

PREP TIME: 5 MINUTES

COOK TIME: ABOUT
10 MINUTES

Substitution Tip: For a soy-free version, substitute coconut aminos for the soy sauce.

PER SERVING

Calories: 270
Protein: 1g
Total Fat: 11g
Saturated Fat: 2g
Carbohydrates: 40g
Fiber: 1g
Sodium: 74mg

This quick noodle dish is bursting with nutty sesame flavor. Feel free to dress it up with additional vegetables—red or yellow bell peppers, diced cucumber, or grated carrots, for instance—or add more fresh herbs, such as mint or basil. Serve alongside barbecued pork, chicken, or prawns.

1 package rice noodles, such as pad Thai noodles

FOR THE SAUCE
¼ cup gluten-free soy sauce
3 tablespoons dark sesame oil
2 tablespoons rice vinegar
2 tablespoons sugar
1 tablespoon Garlic Oil (page 202)
½ teaspoon chili oil or onion- and garlic-free chili paste
2 tablespoons chopped cilantro (optional)

1. Cook the noodles according to the package instructions.

2. While the noodles are cooking, make the sauce. In a small bowl, whisk together the soy sauce, sesame oil, vinegar, sugar, Garlic Oil, and chili oil or paste until well combined.

3. In a large bowl, toss the warm, cooked noodles with the sauce until well coated. Serve immediately, garnished with cilantro if desired.

Crispy Rosemary-Roasted Potatoes

SERVES 6

PREP TIME: 10 MINUTES

COOK TIME: 60 MINUTES

Ingredient Tip: The best roasting potatoes are those with medium amounts of starch, such as Yukon Golds, Yellow Finns, red potatoes, or visually stunning purple potatoes.

PER SERVING

Calories: 106
Protein: 1g
Total Fat: 5g
Saturated Fat: 1g
Carbohydrates: 13g
Fiber: 2g
Sodium: 401mg

Baby potatoes tossed with herbs and olive oil, then baked to a crispy finish, are the perfect accompaniment to roasted or grilled meats, poultry, or fish. If you like, try substituting different fresh herbs, such as thyme, oregano, or sage.

2 pounds small red- or white-skinned new potatoes, halved
2 tablespoons olive oil
2 tablespoons chopped fresh rosemary
1 teaspoon salt

1. Preheat the oven to 400°F.

2. Toss the potatoes, oil, rosemary, and salt together in a large baking dish. Spread the potatoes out in an even layer and roast in the preheated oven for about 60 minutes, until the potatoes are nicely browned and crisp. Serve hot.

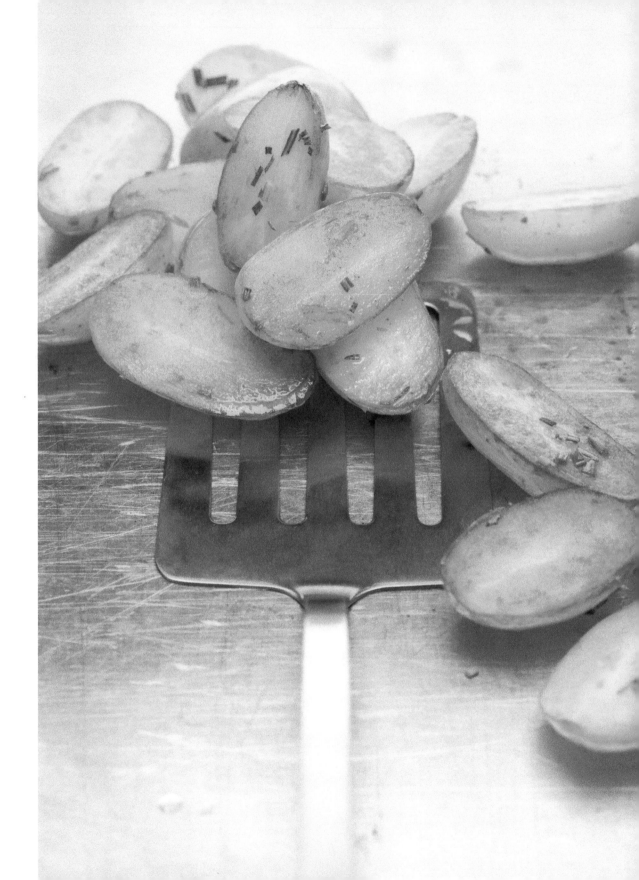

Bacon Mashed Potatoes

SERVES 4

PREP TIME: 10 MINUTES

COOK TIME: 15 MINUTES

Substitution Tip: For a dairy-free version, use rice milk or another nondairy milk instead of the lactose-free milk, and use a vegan butter substitute in place of the butter. You can also crumble in Eggplant Bacon (page 71) to make the dish vegetarian.

PER SERVING

Calories: 203
Protein: 5g
Total Fat: 14g
Saturated Fat: 8g
Carbohydrates: 16g
Fiber: 3g
Sodium: 479mg

Mashed potatoes are always a crowd pleaser. Add bacon, and there's no question that your crowd will gobble them up. This dish is simple and quick to make, but full of flavor. Serve these potatoes alongside roasted meats for a special meal.

1 pound new or baby potatoes, cut into 1-inch cubes
2 slices bacon
⅓ cup lactose-free milk
½ teaspoon salt
¼ teaspoon freshly ground black pepper
¼ cup unsalted butter
4 scallions, green parts only, sliced

1. Put the potatoes in a large saucepan, cover with 2 inches of water, and bring to a boil over medium-high heat. Lower the heat to medium and cook for 10 to 12 minutes, until the potatoes are tender. Drain the potatoes and place them in a large bowl.

2. While the potatoes are cooking, cook the bacon in a large skillet over medium heat for about 4 minutes per side, until browned and crisp. Drain on paper towels, and then crumble.

3. In the large bowl, mash the potatoes with a potato masher. Add the milk, salt, pepper, and butter. Continue mashing until the potatoes are smooth, the butter is melted, and everything is well mixed. Stir in the bacon and scallions. Serve immediately.

Creamy Oven-Baked Polenta with Corn and Parmesan Cheese

SERVES 6

PREP TIME: 5 MINUTES

COOK TIME: 60 MINUTES

Substitution Tip: For a dairy-free version, omit the Parmesan cheese and replace the butter with 2 tablespoons vegan butter substitute or olive oil.

PER SERVING

Calories: 179
Protein: 6g
Total Fat: 6g
Saturated Fat: 4g
Carbohydrates: 26g
Fiber: 1g
Sodium: 508mg

Polenta is a fantastically versatile, gluten-free side dish. This cheesy version is delicious on its own or as an accompaniment to roasted or braised meats. It can also serve as a great base for your favorite pasta sauce.

Oil for preparing the baking dish
1 cup uncooked polenta
3½ cups water
1 cup fresh or frozen corn kernels
1 teaspoon salt
⅓ cup freshly grated Parmesan cheese
2 tablespoons butter

1. Preheat the oven to 350°F.

2. Oil an 8-by-8-inch baking dish. In this dish, stir together the polenta, water, corn, and salt.

3. Bake, uncovered, in the preheated oven for 45 minutes. Stir in the cheese and butter, and bake for an additional 15 minutes. Serve hot.

Quinoa with Swiss Chard

SERVES 4

PREP TIME: 5 MINUTES

COOK TIME: 25 MINUTES

Ingredient Tip: Quinoa should always be rinsed thoroughly before cooking to get rid of its waxy, bitter residue which can upset some stomachs. Use a fine-meshed sieve and cold water for rinsing.

PER SERVING

Calories: 207
Protein: 9g
Total Fat: 7g
Saturated Fat: 1g
Carbohydrates: 29g
Fiber: 4g
Sodium: 753mg

Tender greens, heady spices, and toothsome quinoa make this a satisfying and delicious side dish for meat or fish. To turn it into a meal in and of itself, try topping it with poached eggs and crumbled goat cheese.

1 tablespoon Garlic Oil (page 202)
1 bunch Swiss chard, stems removed and leaves julienned
1 teaspoon ground cumin
1 teaspoon ground coriander
2 teaspoons paprika
½ teaspoon salt
1 cup quinoa
2 cups homemade (onion- and garlic-free) vegetable broth

1. Heat the oil in a large skillet set over medium heat. Add the Swiss chard, cumin, coriander, paprika, salt, quinoa, and broth and bring to a boil.

2. Cover, reduce the heat to low, and cook for 20 minutes, until the liquid has evaporated and the quinoa is tender. Serve hot.

Tomato, Basil, and Olive Risotto

SERVES 4

PREP TIME: 10 MINUTES

COOK TIME: 40 MINUTES

Substitution Tip: For a dairy-free version, replace the butter with a dairy-free butter substitute and omit the Parmesan cheese. Add additional salt if needed.

PER SERVING

Calories: 583
Protein: 44g
Total Fat: 26g
Saturated Fat: 12g
Carbohydrates: 43g
Fiber: 3g
Sodium: 456mg

Risotto takes time to cook, but the process is simple. Hot broth is added to the rice a little at a time so that each addition is absorbed before the next is added. The result is tender, but distinct, grains of plum rice. Here, tomatoes, olives, and fresh basil add flavor and color.

3 cups homemade (onion- and garlic-free) chicken or vegetable broth
3 tablespoons unsalted butter, divided
2 tablespoons olive oil
1 cup Arborio rice
1 (14-ounce) can onion- and garlic-free diced tomatoes, drained
6 Kalamata olives, finely chopped
½ cup chopped fresh basil
¾ cup freshly grated Parmesan cheese

1. In a small saucepan, bring the broth to a boil over medium heat. Reduce the heat to low to maintain a gentle simmer.

2. In a large saucepan, heat 1 tablespoon of the butter and the olive oil over medium heat. Add the rice and stir to coat. Add the tomatoes, olives, and about 1 cup of the broth and cook, stirring constantly, until most of the liquid has been absorbed.

3. Continue adding the broth, one ladleful at time, and cook, stirring frequently, until each addition is fully absorbed, about 30 minutes. When all the liquid has been used up and the rice is tender, remove the pan from the heat and stir in the basil, the remaining butter, and the cheese.

4. Cover the risotto and let rest for about 5 minutes. Serve hot, garnished with additional cheese, if desired.

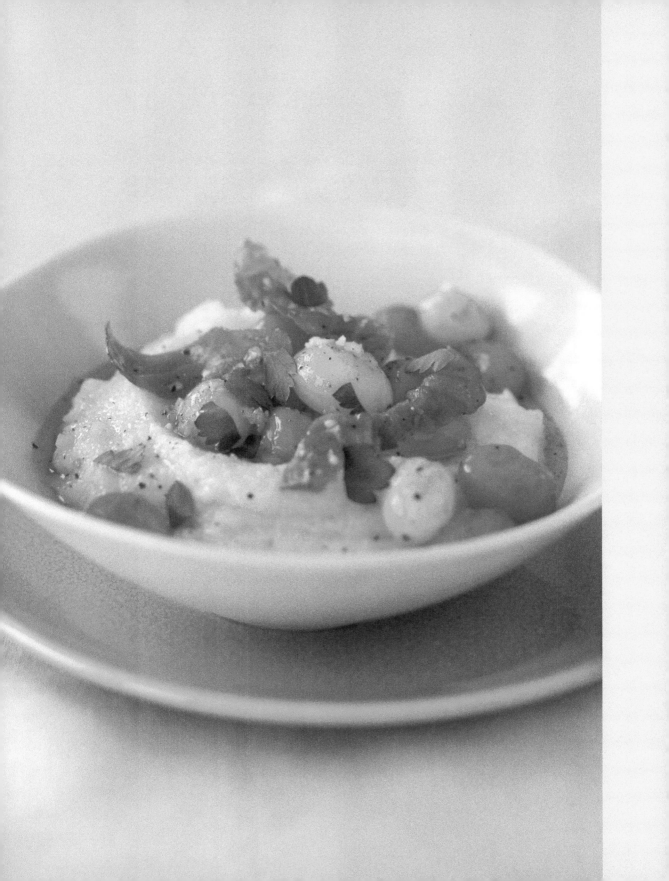

7

Vegetarian and Vegan

Curried Squash Soup with Coconut Milk

SERVES 4

PREP TIME: 10 MINUTES

COOK TIME: 15 MINUTES

Ingredient Tip: When buying pumpkin purée, make sure the product you are buying is 100 percent pure pumpkin and does not contain sweeteners.

PER SERVING

Calories: 155
Protein: 3g
Total Fat: 10g
Saturated Fat: 4g
Carbohydrates: 17g
Fiber: 4g
Sodium: 638mg

This flavorful soup incorporates three different squashes—pattypan, zucchini, and pumpkin—and is flavored with Garlic Oil, fresh ginger, curry powder, and other spices. It takes just a few minutes to whip up, but is incredibly nourishing and satisfying. Serve it with crusty gluten-free rolls or ladle it over cooked rice or quinoa.

1 tablespoon coconut oil
1 tablespoon Garlic Oil (page 202)
1 tablespoon minced fresh ginger
8 pattypan squash, diced
2 medium zucchini, diced
1 teaspoon gluten-free, onion- and garlic-free curry powder
1 teaspoon salt
¾ teaspoon ground coriander
½ teaspoon ground cumin
¼ teaspoon ground cloves
¼ teaspoon cayenne
4 cups homemade (onion- and garlic-free) vegetable broth
½ cup light coconut milk
1 cup pure pumpkin purée
2 tablespoons chopped fresh cilantro, for garnish

1. Heat the coconut oil and Garlic Oil in a stockpot over medium-high heat. Add the ginger and cook for 1 minute. Add the pattypan squash and zucchini, and cook, stirring frequently, until the squash softens, about 3 minutes. Stir in the curry powder, salt, coriander, cumin, cloves, and cayenne, and cook, stirring, for 1 minute more. Add the broth, coconut milk, and pumpkin purée, and bring to a boil. Reduce the heat to low and simmer for about 10 minutes.

2. Purée the soup either in a blender in batches or in the pot using an immersion blender. Return to the heat if needed and heat through.

3. Serve hot, garnished with cilantro.

Smoky Corn Chowder with Red Peppers

SERVES 4

PREP TIME: 10 MINUTES

COOK TIME: 45 MINUTES

Ingredient Tip: Fresh corn is moderately high in FODMAPs, though half a cob per person is usually okay for most people. To be on the safe side, use canned corn for this recipe; canning causes water-soluble FODMAPs to leach into the water, thereby lowering the overall FODMAP quantity.

PER SERVING

Calories: 355
Protein: 13g
Total Fat: 7g
Saturated Fat: 1g
Carbohydrates: 69g
Fiber: 8g
Sodium: 1416mg

This vegan chowder gets its thickness from potatoes, its creaminess from rice milk, and its sweet and spicy flavor from smoked paprika and other spices.

1 tablespoon olive oil
1 tablespoon Garlic Oil (page 202)
1 (10-inch) stalk celery, diced
2 carrots, diced
1 leek (green part only),
   halved lengthwise and thinly sliced
2 red bell peppers, seeded and diced
4 Yukon Gold potatoes, diced (about 1 pound)
2 cups canned corn kernels, divided
4 cups homemade (onion- and garlic-free) vegetable broth
1 teaspoon ground cumin
½ teaspoon smoked paprika
⅛ teaspoon cayenne
1 teaspoon salt
1 cup rice milk
3 scallions, green parts only, thinly sliced

1. Heat the olive oil and Garlic Oil in a stockpot over medium heat. Add the celery and carrots and cook, stirring occasionally, for about 5 minutes, until the vegetables begin to soften. Add the leek, red bell peppers, potatoes, 1 cup of the corn, broth, cumin, smoked paprika, cayenne, and salt, and bring to a boil. Reduce the heat to low and simmer for about 30 minutes, until the potatoes are very tender.

2. Using an immersion blender or in batches in a countertop blender, purée the soup.

3. Stir in the remaining cup of corn and the rice milk, and cook over low heat for about 10 minutes more, until the soup is heated through and the corn kernels are tender. Serve immediately, garnished with sliced scallions.

Kale-Pesto Soba Noodles

SERVES 4

PREP TIME: 10 MINUTES

COOK TIME: 10 MINUTES

Substitution Tip: For a dairy-free version, omit the Parmesan cheese and substitute ½ cup nutritional yeast.

PER SERVING

Calories: 922
Protein: 26g
Total Fat: 68g
Saturated Fat: 11g
Carbohydrates: 67g
Fiber: 4g
Sodium: 1293mg

Traditionally, soba noodles are made of buckwheat (which is not a type of wheat, but a different grain altogether), so they are naturally gluten free (note that not all brands of soba noodles available are made from 100 percent buckwheat, so be sure to check the label). Here they're tossed with a pesto made with lemon juice and fresh kale leaves for a flavorful Italian-Japanese fusion dish that is sure to satisfy.

1 (10-ounce) package gluten-free soba noodles
4 cups kale, removed from stems and roughly chopped
Zest and juice of 1 lemon
1 cup pine nuts
¾ cup grated Parmesan cheese, plus more for serving
¾ cup olive oil
2 tablespoons Garlic Oil (page 202)
¾ teaspoon salt
½ teaspoon freshly ground black pepper

1. Cook the soba noodles according to the instructions on the package.

2. While the noodles are cooking, prepare the pesto. In a food processor, combine the kale, lemon zest and juice, pine nuts, and cheese, and pulse until the kale is finely chopped. With the processor running, slowly add the olive oil in a thin stream, and continue to process to a smooth purée. Add the Garlic Oil, salt, and pepper, and pulse to combine.

3. When the noodles are finished cooking, drain them and immediately toss them with the pesto. Serve immediately, garnished with additional cheese, if desired.

Vegan Noodles with Gingered Coconut Sauce

SERVES 4

PREP TIME: 10 MINUTES

COOK TIME: 10 MINUTES

Substitution Tip: Feel free to substitute kale or broccoli for the chard or spinach, if desired.

PER SERVING

Calories: 569
Protein: 11g
Total Fat: 15g
Saturated Fat: 1g
Carbohydrates: 99g
Fiber: 8g
Sodium: 908mg

The rich coconut milk–based sauce spiked with fresh ginger gets a bright green hue—along with plenty of flavor and nutrition—from fresh chard and baby spinach leaves. Serve it with a side of grilled tofu, chicken, or fish.

1 tablespoon Garlic Oil (page 202)
2½ tablespoons minced fresh ginger
1 (15-ounce) can light coconut milk
2 teaspoons sugar
2 teaspoons lemon juice
1 teaspoon salt
½ teaspoon freshly ground black pepper
Red pepper flakes, to taste
1 bunch of Swiss chard leaves, thick center stems removed, leaves julienned
2 cups baby spinach
1 (16-ounce) package gluten-free spaghetti, cooked al dente according to package directions and drained
2 tablespoons chopped fresh basil

1. Heat the Garlic Oil in a large sauté pan over medium heat. Add the ginger and cook, stirring, for about 3 minutes. Stir in the coconut milk, sugar, lemon juice, salt, pepper, and red pepper flakes and bring just to a boil. Reduce the heat to medium low and add the chard and spinach to the simmering sauce. Cook, stirring occasionally, until the greens are completely wilted, about 5 minutes.

2. Transfer the sauce mixture to a blender and purée, or transfer it to a bowl and purée it using an immersion blender.

3. Return the puréed sauce to the pan and bring it back to a simmer over medium heat. Add the prepared noodles and cook, stirring, until heated through, about 2 to 3 minutes. Serve immediately, garnished with basil.

Baked Tofu *Báhn Mì* Lettuce Wrap

SERVES 4

PREP TIME: 45 MINUTES
TO DRAIN AND MARINATE
TOFU, AND 20 MINUTES TO
PICKLE VEGETABLES

COOK TIME: 20 MINUTES

Substitution Tip: For a
soy-free version, substi-
tute grilled zucchini or
eggplant strips for
the tofu.

PER SERVING

Calories: 180
Protein: 6g
Total Fat: 3g
Saturated Fat: 0g
Carbohydrates: 28g
Fiber: 2g
Sodium: 4138mg

Technically báhn mì *refers to the crusty, baguette-like rolls used to make the traditional Vietnamese sandwiches—loaded with pickled vegetables, chiles, and fresh herbs—of the same name. Here we've packed all of those scrumptious flavors into lettuce leaves, but you could substitute gluten-free baguettes if you prefer.*

FOR THE TOFU
1 (16-ounce) package firm tofu, drained and cut into
   ½-inch-thick slabs
2 tablespoons gluten-free soy sauce
2 teaspoons grated fresh ginger
Vegetable oil or coconut oil to prepare the baking sheet

FOR THE VEGETABLES
½ cup rice vinegar
¼ cup water
¼ cup sugar
1 teaspoon salt
1½ cups shredded carrot
1½ cups shredded daikon radish

FOR THE WRAPS
8 large lettuce leaves
2 tablespoons mayonnaise
½ medium cucumber, peeled, seeded, and cut into matchsticks
2 large jalapeño chiles, thinly sliced
1 cup cilantro leaves

1. Line a rimmed baking sheet with paper towels and place the cut tofu on the sheet in a single layer. Top with another layer of paper towels and then another baking sheet. Weight the top baking sheet down with something heavy (cans of tomatoes or beans work well). Let sit for 30 minutes.

2. While the tofu is draining, prepare the vegetables. In a small saucepan, combine the vinegar, water, sugar, and salt and cook, stirring, over medium heat, until the sugar has dissolved, for about 3 minutes. Remove the pan from the heat and add the carrot and daikon, stirring to coat well. Let sit for 20 minutes.

3. In a large bowl, combine the soy sauce and ginger. Add the pressed tofu and toss to coat well.

4. Let the tofu sit for about 15 minutes, and preheat the oven to 350°F.

5. Oil a large baking sheet with vegetable or coconut oil.

6. Arrange the tofu slabs in a single layer on the prepared baking sheet and bake in the preheated oven for about 10 minutes. Turn the pieces over and bake for another 10 minutes, until the tofu is browned. Remove from the oven and cut into 1-inch-wide sticks.

7. To make the wraps, arrange the lettuce leaves on your work surface and spread a bit of mayonnaise on each, dividing equally. Fill with the baked tofu, cucumber, chiles, and cilantro. Drain the pickled carrots and daikon, and place a handful onto each wrap. Serve immediately.

Roasted-Veggie Gyros with Tzatziki Sauce

SERVES 4

PREP TIME: 15 MINUTES

COOK TIME: 35 MINUTES

Substitution Tip: For
a dairy-free version,
substitute plain, cultured
coconut yogurt for the
lactose-free yogurt.

PER SERVING

Calories: 342
Protein: 14g
Total Fat: 15g
Saturated Fat: 2g
Carbohydrates: 46g
Fiber: 12g
Sodium: 1023mg

Filled with succulent roasted vegetables and a tangy, herby tzatziki sauce, these gluten-free wraps make a delicious lunch or light dinner. Serve with a classic Greek salad on the side.

FOR THE ROASTED VEGETABLES

1 large zucchini, chopped into half moons
1 large yellow squash, chopped into half moons
1 large eggplant, cut into 1-inch cubes
1 cup cherry tomatoes, halved
¼ cup olive oil
1 tablespoon chopped fresh oregano
1½ teaspoons salt
¾ teaspoon freshly ground black pepper

FOR THE SAUCE

1 medium cucumber, peeled, seeded, coarsely grated and
    squeezed in a clean dish towel to remove excess moisture
8 ounces plain lactose-free yogurt
1 tablespoon Garlic Oil (page 202)
1 tablespoon white-wine vinegar
1 tablespoon chopped fresh dill
1 tablespoon lemon juice

TO SERVE

4 gluten-free pita pockets or gluten-free naan
4 large lettuce leaves

1. Preheat the oven to 425°F.

2. On a large, rimmed baking sheet, toss the zucchini, yellow squash, eggplant, and cherry tomatoes together with the olive oil, oregano, salt, and pepper. Spread the vegetables out in an even layer and roast in the preheated oven for about 35 minutes, until they are soft and browned.

3. While the vegetables are roasting, make the sauce. In a medium bowl, combine the cucumber, yogurt, Garlic Oil, vinegar, dill, and lemon juice, and stir to combine. Refrigerate, covered, until ready to serve.

4. Wrap the pitas in foil and heat in the oven (you can place them in the oven along with the vegetables while they're roasting) for about 10 minutes.

5. To serve, fill each pita with the roasted vegetables, top with a dollop of the tzatziki sauce, and garnish each with a lettuce leaf. Serve immediately.

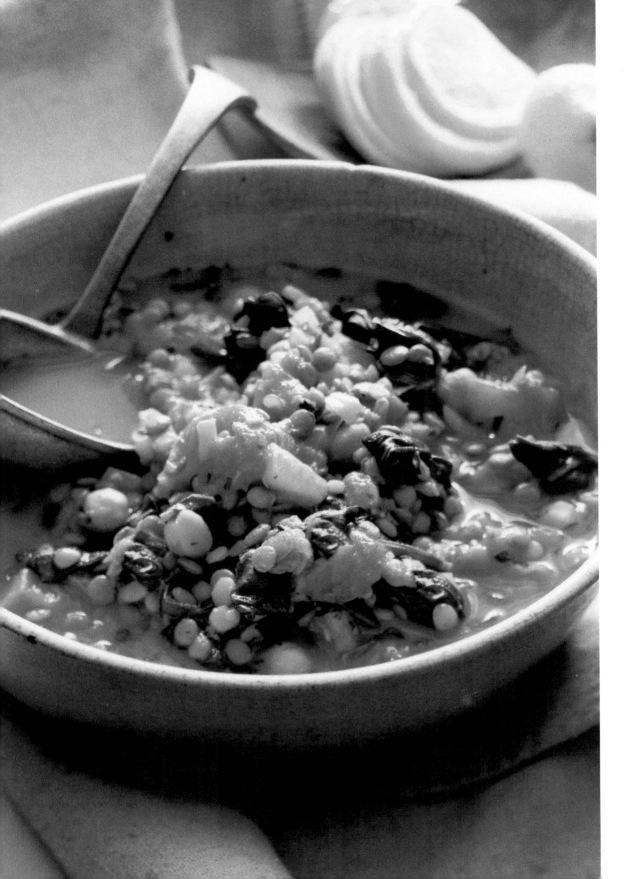

Moroccan-Spiced Lentil and Quinoa Stew

SERVES 4

PREP TIME: 10 MINUTES

COOK TIME: 30 MINUTES

Cooking Tip: To make a "brothier" version of this recipe—more of a soup than a stew—simply leave out the quinoa.

PER SERVING

Calories: 638
Protein: 43g
Total Fat: 11g
Saturated Fat: 2g
Carbohydrates: 97g
Fiber: 36g
Sodium: 2541mg

This spicy lentil stew offers a welcome, hearty meal on a cold winter night. It keeps well in the refrigerator or freezer, so make a big pot and store it in individual servings to have a satisfying meal at the ready. If you like, top it with a dollop of soy or cultured coconut yogurt.

1 tablespoon olive oil
4 carrots, diced
1 leek (green part only), halved lengthwise and thinly sliced
1 tablespoon Garlic Oil (page 202)
1 teaspoon ground cumin
1 teaspoon ground coriander
1 teaspoon ground turmeric
¼ teaspoon ground cinnamon
1½ teaspoons salt
¼ teaspoon freshly ground black pepper
8 cups homemade (onion- and garlic-free) vegetable broth
¾ cup uncooked quinoa, rinsed
1¾ cups canned lentils
1 (28-ounce) can onion- and garlic-free diced tomatoes, drained
2 tablespoons tomato paste
4 cups chopped fresh spinach or 1 (10-ounce) package frozen chopped spinach, thawed
½ cup chopped fresh cilantro
2 tablespoons lemon juice

1. Heat the olive oil in a medium stockpot set over medium heat. Add the carrots and leek, and cook, stirring frequently, for about 10 minutes, until the carrots soften. Add the Garlic Oil, cumin, coriander, turmeric, cinnamon, salt, and pepper. Cook, stirring, for about 1 minute more. ▶

2. Stir in the broth, quinoa, lentils, tomatoes, and tomato paste, and bring the mixture to a boil. Reduce the heat to low and simmer, stirring occasionally, for about 20 minutes, until the quinoa is tender.

3. Stir in the spinach and cook for 5 minutes more.

4. Stir in the cilantro and lemon juice, and serve immediately.

Watercress Zucchini Soup

SERVES 4

PREP TIME: 10 MINUTES

COOK TIME: 15 MINUTES

Cooking Tip: If you wish, you can replace the watercress with chopped fresh spinach.

PER SERVING

Calories: 161
Total Fat: 11g
Saturated Fat: 3g
Cholesterol: 10mg
Carbohydrates: 9g
Fiber: 2g
Protein: 7g

This delicious watercress and zucchini soup is packed with antioxidants including vitamin A and vitamin C. To make the soup, puree it in a food processor or blender before adding the cream at the end. To make it allergen-free, substitute coconut milk.

2 tablespoons extra-virgin olive oil

1 leek, white part removed and the greens finely chopped

3 cups homemade (onion- and garlic-free) vegetable broth

1 pound zucchini, chopped

8 ounces chopped watercress

2 tablespoons dried tarragon

1 teaspoon salt

¼ teaspoon freshly ground black pepper

2 tablespoons heavy cream

1. In a large pot, heat the olive oil over medium-high heat until it shimmers.

2. Add the leek greens and cook, stirring occasionally, until the vegetables are soft, about seven minutes.

3. Add the vegetable broth and zucchini and simmer, stirring occasionally, for eight minutes.

4. Add the watercress, tarragon, salt, and pepper. Cook, stirring occasionally, an additional five minutes.

5. Carefully transfer the soup mixture to a blender or food processor. You may need to work in batches. ▶

6. Fold a towel and place it over the top of the blender with your hand on top of it. Puree the soup for 30 seconds, and then remove the lid to vent steam. Close the blender and puree for another 30 seconds, until the mixture is smooth.

7. Transfer the mixture back to the cooking pot and stir in the heavy cream. Serve immediately.

Lentil-Walnut Burgers

SERVES 6

PREP TIME: 15 MINUTES,
PLUS 1 HOUR FOR
REFRIGERATION

COOK TIME: 10 MINUTES

Substitution Tip: For a
nut-free version, substi-
tute ½ cup mashed
chickpeas for the walnuts.

PER SERVING

Calories: 292
Protein: 13g
Total Fat: 6g
Saturated Fat: 1g
Carbohydrates: 48g
Fiber: 7g
Sodium: 764mg

These vegetarian burger patties are a great alternative to meat-based versions. Serve them any way you'd serve a classic burger, with basic burger toppings like tomato, lettuce, and mustard, or with cheese, salsa, guacamole, or barbecue sauce.

1½ cups canned lentils, rinsed and drained
1 tablespoon homemade (onion- and garlic-free)
   vegetable broth or water
2 teaspoons olive oil
8 ounces fresh baby spinach
Juice of ½ lemon
1 teaspoon salt, divided
½ teaspoon freshly ground black pepper
½ teaspoon ground cumin
1 cup gluten-free bread crumbs
½ cup walnuts, toasted and finely chopped
Cooking spray

TO SERVE
6 gluten-free hamburger buns
2 cups baby arugula
1 large tomato, sliced
2 tablespoons spicy mustard

1. In a medium bowl, mash the lentils with a potato masher, adding the tablespoon of broth or water.

2. Heat the oil in a large skillet set over medium heat. Add the spinach, lemon juice, ¼ teaspoon of the salt, pepper, and cumin and cook, stirring, until the spinach is cooked, about 3 minutes. ▶

Lentil-Walnut Burgers *continued*

3. Add the spinach mixture, bread crumbs, walnuts, and the remaining ¾ teaspoon of salt to the mashed lentils, and stir to mix well. Refrigerate, covered, for at least 1 hour.

4. Coat a grill or grill pan with cooking spray and heat it to medium-high heat. Shape the lentil mixture into six patties, each about 4 inches across. Cook the patties for about 3 minutes on each side, until grill marks appear. Serve the patties hot on gluten-free buns, garnished with arugula, tomato, and spicy mustard.

Zucchini Pasta alla Puttanesca

SERVES 4

PREP TIME: 10 MINUTES

COOK TIME: 15 MINUTES

Substitution Tip: For a dairy-free version, omit the Parmesan cheese, and garnish with 2 tablespoons nutritional yeast, if desired.

PER SERVING

Calories: 226
Protein: 14g
Total Fat: 15g
Saturated Fat: 5g
Carbohydrates: 16g
Fiber: 5g
Sodium: 974mg

This light entrée actually includes no pasta at all, just zucchini sliced into long noodles using a spiral slicer and tossed with a fresh, spicy tomato sauce studded with olives and capers. If you prefer a heartier version, substitute gluten-free spaghetti for the zucchini.

2 tablespoons olive oil
1½ cups diced tomatoes
1 tablespoon Garlic Oil (page 202)
2 tablespoons chopped Kalamata olives
1 tablespoon capers, drained
1 teaspoon salt
½ teaspoon freshly ground black pepper
½ teaspoon red pepper flakes
¼ cup chopped fresh basil
3 large zucchini, cut into ribbons with a spiral slicer
½ cup freshly grated Parmesan cheese

1. Heat the olive oil in a large skillet over medium-high heat. Add the tomatoes and Garlic Oil, and cook for about 10 minutes, until the tomatoes begin to break down and become saucy. Add the olives, capers, salt, pepper, and red pepper flakes, and cook for 5 minutes more. Stir in the basil.

2. Remove the pan from the heat and add the zucchini. Toss until the zucchini noodles soften and are well coated with the sauce. Serve immediately, garnished with Parmesan cheese.

Coconut-Curry Tofu with Vegetables

SERVES 4

PREP TIME: 10 MINUTES

COOK TIME: 25 MINUTES

Substitution Tip: For a soy-free version, omit the tofu and include additional vegetables such as broccoli florets, diced zucchini, or butternut squash. Add the vegetables along with the peppers, and increase the cooking time, if needed.

PER SERVING

Calories: 321
Protein: 16g
Total Fat: 25g
Saturated Fat: 14g
Carbohydrates: 17g
Fiber: 6g
Sodium: 756mg

This savory tofu and veggie dish is quick to prepare and, when served over steamed rice or quinoa, makes for a satisfying meal. It's versatile too: Just add or substitute other vegetables you have on hand, such as broccoli, butternut squash, or chard.

FOR THE SAUCE
1 cup canned coconut milk
2 tablespoons chopped fresh cilantro
1 tablespoon gluten-free, onion- and garlic-free curry powder
1 teaspoon brown sugar
1 teaspoon salt

FOR THE TOFU AND VEGETABLES
1 tablespoon grapeseed oil
14 ounces extra-firm tofu, drained and cut into cubes
1 red bell pepper, sliced
1 zucchini, halved lengthwise and sliced
2 cups broccoli florets
1 bunch baby bok choy, cut into 2-inch pieces

1. To make the sauce, in a small bowl, stir together the coconut milk, cilantro, curry powder, brown sugar, and salt.

2. To prepare the tofu and vegetables, heat the oil in a large skillet over high heat. Arrange the tofu in the pan in a single layer and cook, without stirring, for about 5 minutes, until it begins to brown on the bottom. Scrape the tofu from the pan with a spatula and continue to cook, stirring occasionally, until it is golden brown all over, for about 7 more minutes.

3. Add the bell pepper, zucchini, broccoli, and bok choy to the pan, along with the sauce mixture, and continue to cook, stirring, for about 8 to 10 minutes, until the vegetables are tender. Serve immediately.

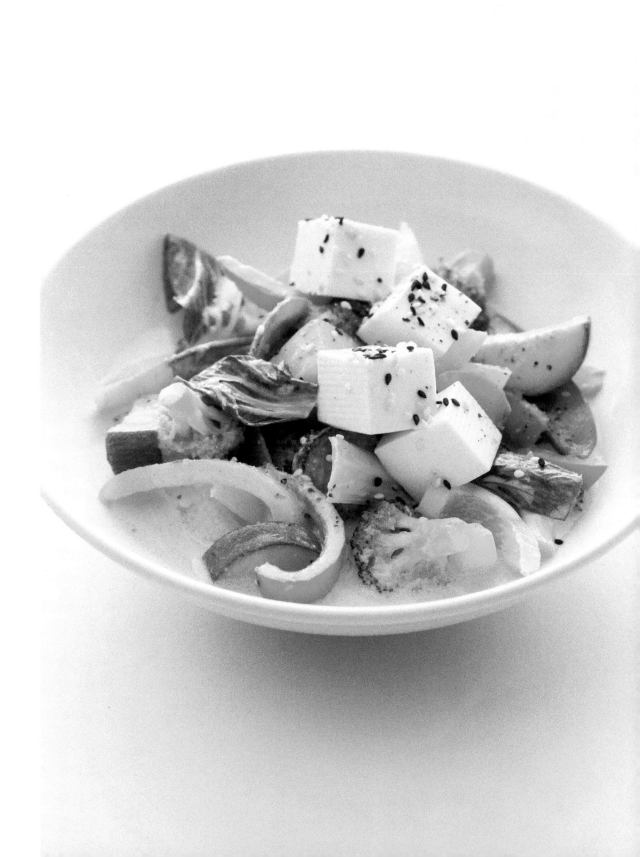

Quinoa-Stuffed Eggplant Roulades with Feta and Mint

SERVES 4

PREP TIME: 15 MINUTES

COOK TIME: 45 MINUTES

Substitution Tip: For a dairy-free version, leave out the cheese and substitute ½ cup chopped olives. For a nut-free version, omit the pine nuts.

PER SERVING

Calories: 422
Protein: 11g
Total Fat: 25g
Saturated Fat: 6g
Carbohydrates: 44g
Fiber: 14g
Sodium: 894mg

Eggplant roulades are easy to assemble, and the finished dish is impressive. This version includes bright, fresh mint leaves and a sprinkling of tangy feta cheese for a bit of Mediterranean flair. Serve it with a classic Greek salad for a filling vegetarian meal.

3 tablespoons olive oil, divided

½ cup uncooked quinoa, rinsed

1 cup water

¼ cup toasted pine nuts

2 medium eggplants, sliced lengthwise into ¼-inch-thick slices

½ teaspoon salt

½ teaspoon freshly ground black pepper

1½ cups onion- and garlic-free tomato sauce or marinara sauce (such as Rao's Sensitive Formula Marinara Sauce)

2 tablespoons chopped fresh mint

½ cup crumbled feta cheese

1. Preheat the oven to 375°F.

2. Grease a large baking dish with 1 tablespoon of the olive oil.

3. In a small saucepan, combine the quinoa and water, and bring to a boil over high heat. Reduce the heat to low, cover, and simmer for about 15 minutes, until the water has evaporated and the quinoa is tender. Stir in the pine nuts.

4. While the quinoa is cooking, prepare the eggplant slices. Heat the remaining 2 tablespoons of olive oil in a large skillet over medium-high heat. Sprinkle the eggplant slices on both sides with salt and pepper, and add them to the pan, cooking in a single layer (you'll need to cook them in batches). Cook for about 3 minutes per side, until golden brown. Transfer the eggplant slices to a plate as they are cooked.

5. To make the roulades, lay an eggplant slice on your work surface and spoon some of the quinoa onto the bottom. Roll the eggplant up into a tube around the filling. Place the rolls as you complete them into a baking dish, and spoon the marinara sauce over the top. Sprinkle the mint and cheese over the roulades, and bake in the preheated oven until they are heated through and the sauce is bubbly, for about 15 minutes.

Chipotle Tofu and Sweet Potato Tacos with Avocado Salsa

SERVES 4

PREP TIME: 10 MINUTES

COOK TIME: 20 MINUTES

Substitution Tip: For a soy-free version, omit the tofu and add 1½ cups of drained and rinsed canned chickpeas, along with the chipotle and other seasonings.

PER SERVING

Calories: 421
Protein: 15g
Total Fat: 18g
Saturated Fat: 3g
Carbohydrates: 55g
Fiber: 10g
Sodium: 229mg

Tacos make for a delicious, casual meal. This version is filled with a sweet-savory combination of succulent tofu and silky sweet potato, flavored with smoky chipotle chiles and garnished with a spicy avocado salsa. Add a dollop of salsa for even more spice.

FOR THE FILLING
2 tablespoons olive oil
2 sweet potatoes, peeled and cut into ½-inch cubes
1 pound firm tofu, diced
½ to 1 teaspoon ground chipotle chiles
2 tablespoons sugar
Juice of 1 lime

FOR THE AVOCADO SALSA
2 tomatoes
½ avocado, diced
¼ serrano chile, diced
Juice of ½ lime
¼ teaspoon salt
2 tablespoons chopped fresh cilantro

TO SERVE
8 soft corn tortillas

1. Heat the olive oil in a large skillet over medium heat. Add the sweet potatoes and cook for about 5 minutes, until the potatoes begin to soften. Add the tofu, chipotle, sugar, and lime juice. Reduce the heat to low and cook, stirring occasionally, until the sweet potatoes are tender, about 15 minutes.

2. Meanwhile, wrap the tortillas in aluminum foil and heat them in a 350°F oven for 10 minutes.

3. To make the avocado salsa, combine the tomatoes, avocado, chile, lime juice, and salt in a medium bowl. Stir in the cilantro.

4. To serve, fill the tortillas with the filliing, dividing equally, and spoon a dollop of avocado salsa on top of each. Serve immediately.

Tempeh Enchiladas with Red Chili Sauce

SERVES 4 TO 6

PREP TIME: 15 MINUTES

COOK TIME: 60 MINUTES

Substitution Tip: For a soy-free version, omit the tempeh and substitute 1 cup of canned chickpeas.

PER SERVING

Calories: 724
Protein: 38g
Total Fat: 35g
Saturated Fat: 12g
Carbohydrates: 76g
Fiber: 15g
Sodium: 998mg

Making your own enchilada sauce is easy and worth the effort, because most commercial sauces contain wheat flour. These hearty enchiladas are filled with a combination of tempeh, corn, and green chiles and topped with your own rich, red enchilada sauce. Bubbling cheese is an optional, but enticing, finishing touch.

FOR THE SAUCE
2 tablespoons grapeseed oil
2 tablespoons gluten-free all-purpose flour
1 tablespoon Garlic Oil (page 202)
¼ cup gluten-free, onion- and garlic-free chili powder
½ teaspoon salt
¼ teaspoon ground cumin
1 tablespoon minced fresh oregano
2 cups homemade (onion- and garlic-free) vegetable broth

FOR THE ENCHILADAS
12 ounces crumbled tempeh
2 cups canned corn kernels
1 (4-ounce) can diced green chiles
10 small corn tortillas
1½ cups shredded sharp white cheddar cheese (optional)

1. To make the sauce, heat the grapeseed oil in a small saucepan over medium-high heat. Whisk in the flour and cook, stirring, for 1 minute. Stir in the Garlic Oil, chili powder, salt, cumin, and oregano. While stirring constantly, gradually add the broth. Bring to a boil, then reduce the heat to low and simmer, stirring occasionally, for 10 to 15 minutes, until the sauce has thickened. Transfer the sauce to a wide, shallow bowl.

2. In a bowl, stir together the crumbled tempeh, corn, and green chiles.

3. To make the enchiladas, spoon about ⅓ cup of the sauce into a 9-by-13-inch baking dish and spread it out over the bottom of the dish. Wrap the tortillas in a clean dish towel and heat them in the microwave on high for about 30 seconds. Dip each tortilla in the sauce to coat it lightly, then spoon about ¼ cup of the tempeh mixture in a line down the center. Roll the tortilla up around the filling. Set the filled tortilla in the prepared baking dish, seam-side down. Repeat with the remaining tortillas and filling.

4. Spoon the remaining sauce over the top, covering all of the tortillas. Sprinkle the cheese over the top, if using, and bake in the preheated oven for about 40 minutes, until heated through and bubbling. Serve immediately.

Polenta with Roasted Vegetables and Spicy Tomato Sauce

SERVES 4

PREP TIME: 15 MINUTES

COOK TIME: 60 MINUTES

Cooking Tip: Leftover polenta will become solid enough to cut with a knife after being refrigerated overnight. Slice it into sticks or cubes, and bake, fry, or grill them until crisp and browned. Then use them for a snack, appetizer, or side dish. Alternatively, if you'd like to serve creamy polenta for a second time, simply add a bit of broth, lactose-free milk, or water to the leftovers. Then warm the mixture in a saucepan, stirring frequently, until it is runny and heated through.

PER SERVING

Calories: 457
Protein: 12g
Total Fat: 24g
Saturated Fat: 10g
Carbohydrates: 53g
Fiber: 8g
Sodium: 2135mg

Polenta is nearly as simple to make as steamed rice: Once the cornmeal has been incorporated into the boiling water, you can cover the pot and pretty much forget about it while you prepare the rest of the meal. Here the creamy cornmeal dish is topped with roasted vegetables and a spicy Mexican-style tomato sauce.

FOR THE POLENTA
Oil for preparing the baking sheet
4 cups water
1 teaspoon salt
1 cup uncooked polenta
2 tablespoons butter or nondairy butter substitute (optional)

FOR THE VEGETABLES *zucchini*
2 medium red bell peppers, seeded and cut into ¼-inch-thick rings
2 cups assorted grape tomatoes
8 pieces oil-packed sun-dried tomatoes, julienned
2 tablespoons olive oil
1 teaspoon salt
1 teaspoon gluten-free, onion- and garlic-free chili powder
4 ounces crumbled queso fresco or feta cheese (optional)

FOR THE SAUCE
2 jalapeño chiles, seeded and diced
1 tablespoon Garlic Oil (page 202)
1 teaspoon salt
1 (14½-ounce) can onion- and garlic-free diced tomatoes, preferably fire-roasted
2 tablespoons chopped fresh flat-leafed parsley

1. Preheat the oven to 475°F.

2. Oil a large, rimmed baking sheet.

3. To make the polenta, combine the water and salt in a large saucepan, and bring to a boil over medium-high heat. While whisking continuously, slowly add the polenta. Reduce the heat to low and cook, whisking continuously, until the polenta becomes thick. Cover the saucepan and cook for about 30 minutes, stirring every once in a while, until the polenta is creamy and no grittiness remains. Just before serving, stir in the butter, if using.

4. In a large bowl, toss the bell peppers, grape tomatoes, and sun-dried tomatoes with the olive oil. Spread the vegetables on the baking sheet in a single layer. Sprinkle with the salt and chili powder. Roast in the preheated oven, stirring once or twice, until the vegetables are tender and starting to brown, for about 25 minutes.

5. Meanwhile, make the sauce. In a blender, combine the chiles, Garlic Oil, and salt, and blend until smooth. Add the tomatoes and pulse to a chunky, smooth texture. Transfer the mixture to a small saucepan and heat over medium heat. Simmer until the sauce is thickened, for about 6 minutes.

6. To serve, spoon some of the polenta into each of 4 serving bowls. Top with some of the roasted vegetables and spoon some of the warm sauce over the top. Sprinkle the cheese on top, if using. Garnish with parsley and serve immediately.

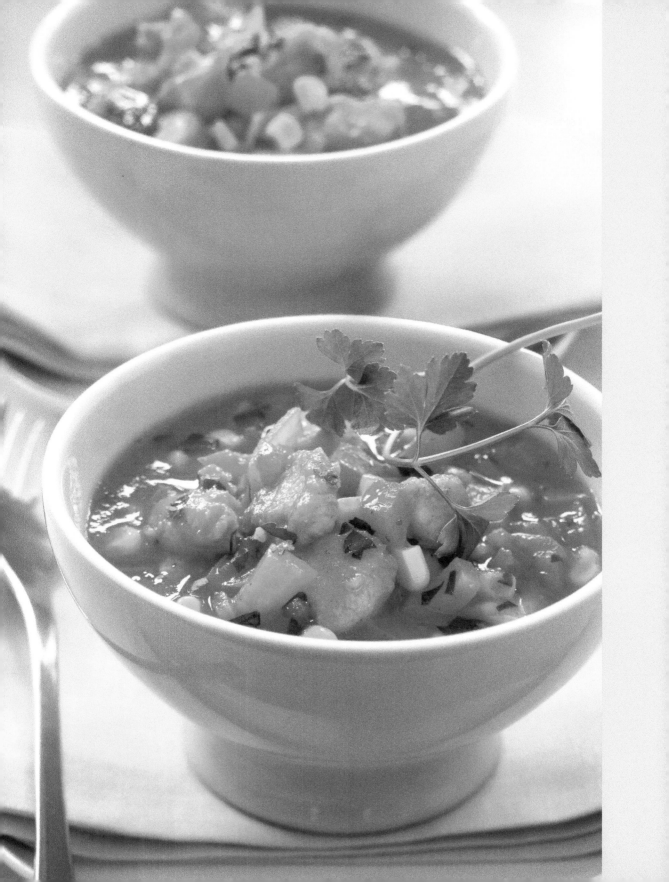

8

Meat and Poultry

Green Chile-Stuffed Turkey Burgers

SERVES 4

PREP TIME: 10 MINUTES

COOK TIME: 15 MINUTES

Substitution Tip: For a soy-free version, substitute coconut aminos for the soy sauce. You can find coconut aminos in the health food aisle of many supermarkets or at a health food store.

PER SERVING

Calories: 501
Protein: 45g
Total Fat: 21g
Saturated Fat: 3g
Carbohydrates: 40g
Fiber: 6g
Sodium: 1481mg

Lighter than classic beef burgers, these turkey burgers are loaded with flavor. They make a great entrée for a backyard cookout, and the recipe is easily doubled, tripled, or quadrupled as needed. If you like, add slices of pepper jack cheese and garnish them with salsa or guacamole.

1¼ pounds ground turkey
2 (4-ounce) cans diced green chiles
2 scallions (green part only), thinly sliced
½ cup chopped fresh cilantro
2 teaspoons ground cumin
1 teaspoon gluten-, onion-, and garlic-free chili powder
1 teaspoon gluten-free soy sauce
1 teaspoon salt
4 gluten-free hamburger buns
4 leaves crisp lettuce, such as Romaine
1 large tomato, sliced
2 tablespoons Dijon mustard
Oil, for preparing the grill

1. In a medium bowl, combine the turkey, chiles, scallions, cilantro, cumin, chili powder, soy sauce, and salt.

2. Form the mixture into 4 patties, about 4 inches across.

3. Oil a grill or grill pan and heat to medium-high heat.

4. Grill the burgers for 5 to 6 minutes per side, until grill marks appear and the burgers are cooked through.

5. Serve the burgers on gluten-free buns with lettuce, tomato slices, and Dijon mustard.

Turkey and Sweet Potato Chili

SERVES 4

PREP TIME: 10 MINUTES

COOK TIME: 30 MINUTES

Cooking Tip: You can make this chili in a slow cooker, if you like. Brown the turkey and add the spices as directed above, then transfer the cooked turkey to the slow cooker, add the bell pepper, tomatoes, chiles, corn, tomato sauce, water, and sweet potato. Cover the slow cooker and cook on high for 4 hours or on low for 6 hours.

PER SERVING

Calories: 390
Protein: 44g
Total Fat: 16g
Saturated Fat: 3g
Carbohydrates: 29g
Fiber: 6g
Sodium: 1326mg

A big pot of chili is the perfect thing to serve on a chilly fall day, whether for a family dinner, a big-game party, or a potluck. This version features sweet potatoes and lots of spices instead of high-FODMAP beans. Serve a gluten-free cornbread alongside for dipping, if you like.

2 tablespoons Garlic Oil (page 202)
1¼ pounds ground turkey
1 red bell pepper, chopped
1 teaspoon salt
½ teaspoon ground cumin
¼ teaspoon gluten-, onion-, and garlic-free chili powder
¼ teaspoon paprika
1 bay leaf
1 (14½-ounce) can onion- and garlic-free diced tomatoes with juice
1 (4-ounce) can diced green chiles
1 cup canned corn, drained and rinsed
1 cup onion- and garlic-free tomato sauce
¾ cup water
1 sweet potato, peeled and diced into ½-inch cubes
2 tablespoons chopped fresh cilantro

1. Heat the Garlic Oil in a large skillet over medium-high heat. Add the turkey and cook, stirring and breaking up the meat with a spatula, until it is browned, for about 5 minutes. Add the bell pepper and cook until it begins to soften, about 3 minutes more.

2. Add the salt, cumin, chili powder, paprika, and bay leaf and cook, stirring, for 1 minute. Add the tomatoes with their juice, chiles, corn, tomato sauce, water, and sweet potato, and bring to a boil. Reduce the heat to low, cover, and simmer for about 25 minutes, stirring occasionally, until the sweet potatoes are tender.

3. Serve hot, garnished with cilantro.

Roasted Chicken, Potatoes, and Kale

SERVES 8

PREP TIME: 10 MINUTES

COOK TIME: 50 MINUTES

Cooking Tip: Using separated drumsticks and thighs makes it easier to serve bigger or smaller portions as needed, but for a more dramatic presentation, use whole chicken legs, with the drumstick and thigh still attached.

PER SERVING

Calories: 458
Protein: 36g
Total Fat: 25g
Saturated Fat: 6g
Carbohydrates: 24g
Fiber: 3g
Sodium: 884mg

This simple one-dish meal makes enough to serve a crowd with very little effort. The potatoes and chicken skin become nicely crisp and golden brown, while a heavenly smell fills your kitchen. Don't skip the squeeze of fresh lemon juice at the end; it takes this dish from good to great.

1½ pounds Yukon Gold potatoes, cut into ¼-inch-thick slices
1½ pounds kale, stems and inner ribs removed
¼ cup olive oil
2 teaspoons salt, divided
½ teaspoon freshly ground black pepper
8 chicken drumsticks
8 chicken thighs
1 teaspoon paprika
Juice of 1 lemon

1. Preheat the oven to 450°F.

2. In a large roasting pan, combine the potatoes and kale, and toss with the olive oil. Spread the vegetables out in an even layer and sprinkle with the pepper and 1 teaspoon of the salt.

3. Season the chicken pieces all over with the remaining teaspoon of salt and arrange them on top of the vegetables in the roasting pan. Sprinkle the paprika over the top, and cover the roasting pan with aluminum foil.

4. Roast the chicken in the preheated oven for 20 minutes. Remove the foil and continue to cook for another 30 minutes, until the chicken is thoroughly cooked and the potatoes are tender. Remove from the oven and let rest for a few minutes before serving.

5. Just before serving, squeeze the lemon over the chicken and vegetables. Serve immediately.

Grilled Chicken with Maple-Mustard Glaze

SERVES 4

PREP TIME: 10 MINUTES,
PLUS 30 MINUTES
TO MARINATE

COOK TIME: 20 MINUTES

Substitution Tip: For a
soy-free version, use
coconut aminos in place
of the soy sauce.

PER SERVING

Calories: 357
Protein: 51g
Total Fat: 8g
Saturated Fat: 3g
Carbohydrates: 16g
Fiber: 0g
Sodium: 879mg

Flavored with tangy mustard and sweet maple syrup, this simple grilled chicken dish will get rave reviews from the whole family. Marinating takes only 30 minutes, but the longer you marinate, the more flavorful the chicken will be. Serve it alongside Classic Coleslaw (page 106) or a crisp green salad.

½ cup onion- and garlic-free spicy brown mustard
2 tablespoons brown sugar
3 tablespoons maple syrup
1 tablespoon white-wine vinegar
2 teaspoons gluten-free soy sauce
½ teaspoon pepper
1 tablespoon Garlic Oil (page 202)
8 skinless, bone-in chicken thighs
Cooking spray
½ teaspoon salt

1. In a small bowl, stir together the mustard, brown sugar, maple syrup, vinegar, soy sauce, pepper, and Garlic Oil. Place the chicken pieces in a resealable plastic bag, and add half of the mustard mixture.

2. Seal the bag and shake to coat the chicken pieces well. Marinate for at least 30 minutes (or up to 2 hours).

3. Spray a grill or grill pan with cooking spray, and heat to medium-high.

4. Remove the chicken pieces from the marinade, discarding the marinade, and sprinkle them with salt. Cook the chicken on the grill until grill marks appear and the chicken is thoroughly cooked, for about 8 minutes per side. Serve immediately, drizzled with the reserved mustard mixture.

Chicken Enchiladas

SERVES 8

PREP TIME: 15 MINUTES

COOK TIME: 45 MINUTES

Substitution Tip: For a dairy-free version, simply omit the cheese or use a dairy-free cheese in its place.

PER SERVING

Calories: 415
Protein: 37g
Total Fat: 13g
Saturated Fat: 3g
Carbohydrates: 41g
Fiber: 9g
Sodium: 759mg

Shredded chicken mixed with corn and chiles makes a succulent filling for enchiladas. You can use a leftover roasted chicken or store-bought rotisserie chicken for the enchilada filling, which makes this a quick dish to put together, even when you make your own sauce from scratch.

FOR THE SAUCE
2 tablespoons grapeseed oil
2 tablespoons gluten-free all-purpose flour
1 tablespoon Garlic Oil (page 202)
¼ cup gluten-, onion-, and garlic-free chili powder
½ teaspoon salt
¼ teaspoon ground cumin
1 tablespoon minced fresh oregano
2 cups homemade (onion- and garlic-free) chicken broth

FOR THE ENCHILADAS
Oil for preparing the baking sheet
1½ pounds cooked, shredded chicken breast (boneless, skinless)
1 cup fresh or frozen (thawed) corn kernels
1 (4-ounce) can diced green chiles
1 teaspoon ground chipotle
1 (14-ounce) can onion- and garlic-free diced tomatoes, drained
½ teaspoon salt
16 corn tortillas
1 cup shredded cheddar or Monterey Jack cheese
¼ cup chopped fresh cilantro

1. To make the sauce, heat the grapeseed oil in a small saucepan over medium-high heat. Whisk in the flour and cook, stirring, for 1 minute. Stir in the Garlic Oil, chili powder, salt, cumin, and oregano. While stirring constantly, gradually add the broth. Bring to a boil, then reduce the heat to low and simmer, stirring occasionally, for 10 to 15 minutes, until the sauce has thickened. Transfer the sauce to a large, shallow bowl.

2. To make the enchiladas, begin by preheating the oven to 350°F.

3. Oil a 9-by-13-inch baking dish.

4. In a large bowl, combine the chicken, corn, green chiles, ground chipotle, tomatoes, and salt, and stir to mix well. Wrap the tortillas in a clean dish towel, and microwave them on high for about 30 seconds.

5. Coat the bottom of the prepared baking dish with several spoonfuls of the sauce. Dip each tortilla in the sauce to coat it lightly. Spoon about ¼ cup of the chicken mixture into the tortilla in a line down the center. Roll the tortilla up around the filling and place it in the prepared baking dish, seam-side down. Repeat with the remaining tortillas and filling. When all of the tortillas are filled and in the baking dish, spoon the remaining sauce over the top, covering all of the tortillas. Sprinkle with the cheese.

6. Bake the enchiladas in the preheated oven until the sauce is bubbly and the cheese is melted, for 15 to 20 minutes. Serve hot, garnished with cilantro.

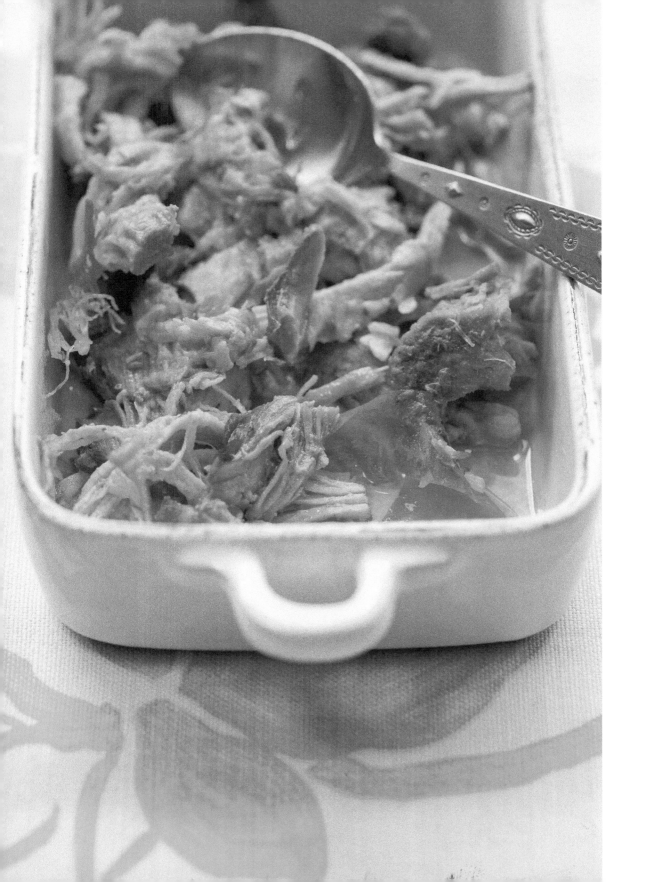

Spicy Pulled Pork

SERVES 8

PREP TIME: 15 MINUTES, PLUS 1 HOUR TO MARINATE

COOK TIME: 6 HOURS

Cooking Tip: If you don't want to tie up your oven all day or won't be around to keep an eye on the pork, make this dish in a slow cooker instead. Rub the meat with the spice mixture, then place it in the slow cooker along with 1 cup of chicken broth. Cover and cook on low for about 10 hours, until the meat is falling apart.

PER SERVING

Calories: 988
Protein: 72g
Total Fat: 67g
Saturated Fat: 23g
Carbohydrates: 20g
Fiber: 4g
Sodium: 3167mg

Whipping up a big batch of this crave-worthy meat is so simple that it's the perfect thing to serve on game day or bring to a potluck. Serve this saucy, spicy, tender meat wrapped in corn tortillas or piled on gluten-free buns. Or for an irresistible sandwich experience, top it with Classic Coleslaw (page 106), the ideal accompaniment.

FOR THE PORK
3 tablespoons paprika
1 tablespoon brown sugar
1 tablespoon dry mustard
3 tablespoons salt
1 pork shoulder or butt roast (about 5 pounds)

FOR THE SAUCE
1½ cups white-wine vinegar
1 cup onion- and garlic-free mustard
⅓ cup onion- and garlic-free tomato sauce
½ cup packed brown sugar
1 tablespoon Garlic Oil (page 202)
1 teaspoon salt
1 teaspoon cayenne
½ teaspoon freshly ground black pepper

1. To prepare the roast, in a small bowl, combine the paprika, brown sugar, dry mustard, and salt.

2. Rub the spice blend all over the pork. Cover and refrigerate for at least 1 hour or as long as overnight.

3. Preheat the oven to 300°F.

4. Roast the pork in a roasting pan in the preheated oven for 6 hours, until the meat is falling apart (a meat thermometer should read about 170°F). ▶

5. While the pork is in the oven, prepare the sauce. In a medium saucepan, combine the vinegar, mustard, tomato sauce, brown sugar, Garlic Oil, salt, cayenne, and black pepper, and bring to a simmer over medium heat. Cook, stirring occasionally, until the sugar is completely dissolved, for about 10 minutes. Remove from the heat.

6. When the pork is done, remove it from the oven and let it rest for about 10 minutes. While the pork is still warm, shred the meat using two forks. Place the shredded meat in a large bowl and mix in half of the sauce.

7. Serve warm, topped with additional sauce.

Arroz con Pollo with Olives, Raisins, and Pine Nuts

SERVES 6 TO 8

PREP TIME: 15 MINUTES,
PLUS 1 HOUR TO MARINATE

COOK TIME: 60 MINUTES

Ingredient Tip: This dish is very forgiving on what type of chicken you use. For instance, you can purchase a whole chicken and have your butcher cut it up for you, you can purchase a pre-packaged cut-up chicken, or you can substitute an equivalent quantity of chicken pieces (e.g., 8 thighs, or 4 thighs and 4 legs).

PER SERVING

Calories: 651
Protein: 55g
Total Fat: 23g
Saturated Fat: 5g
Carbohydrates: 53g
Fiber: 3g
Sodium: 1725mg

Arroz con pollo is a classic comfort food in many Latin cuisines and cultures. This unusual version combines several of these traditions, obtaining both flavor and color from saffron, a common ingredient in Spanish cooking, as well as including plump raisins, briny olives, and crunchy pine nuts.

FOR THE CHICKEN

2 tablespoons orange juice
2 tablespoons lime juice
1½ teaspoons salt
¾ teaspoon freshly ground black pepper
1 whole chicken (about 3½ to 4½ pounds), cut into 8 serving pieces
1 tablespoon vegetable oil
1 tablespoon unsalted butter

FOR THE RICE

2 green bell peppers, diced
¼ teaspoon saffron threads, soaked in ¼ cup warm water
2 teaspoons ground cumin
2 teaspoons salt
1 bay leaf
1 (14½-ounce) can diced onion- and garlic-free tomatoes with juice
1½ cups homemade (onion- and garlic-free) chicken broth
1¼ cups water
1½ cups long-grain white rice
½ cup golden raisins
½ cup small pimiento-stuffed green olives, rinsed
¼ cup toasted pine nuts (optional)

1. To prepare the chicken, combine the orange juice, lime juice, salt, and pepper in a large bowl. Add the chicken and turn to coat. Cover and marinate in the refrigerator for at least 1 hour. ▶

Arroz con Pollo with Olives, Raisins, and Pine Nuts *continued*

2. Remove the chicken from the marinade, reserving the marinade. Pat the chicken pieces dry with paper towels.

3. Heat the oil and butter in a large Dutch oven or stockpot over medium-high heat. Brown the chicken in batches for about 6 minutes per batch, until the chicken is browned on both sides. Transfer the browned chicken pieces to a large plate.

4. To make the rice, begin by preheating the oven to 350°F.

5. Add the bell peppers to the Dutch oven and sauté over medium-high heat, stirring occasionally, until the vegetables soften, for about 8 minutes. Add the saffron along with its soaking liquid, the cumin, salt, bay leaf, tomatoes along with their juice, broth, water, and the reserved marinade. Bring to a boil. Add the chicken pieces except for the breasts. Reduce the heat to low, cover, and simmer for 10 minutes. Stir in the rice and add the chicken breasts, skin-side up, on top of the rice and vegetables. Cover and transfer to the preheated oven. Cook for 20 minutes, until the rice is tender and the liquid has been absorbed.

6. Remove the pot from the oven and sprinkle the raisins, olives, and pine nuts (if using) over the top. Cover the pot with a clean dish towel and let rest for 5 to 10 minutes. Discard the bay leaf.

Italian-Herbed Chicken Meatballs in Broth

SERVES 4

PREP TIME: 15 MINUTES

COOK TIME: 25 MINUTES

Substitution Tip: For a dairy-free version, substitute ⅓ cup nutritional yeast for the Parmesan cheese in the meatballs, and garnish with additional nutritional yeast if desired.

PER SERVING

Calories: 493
Protein: 48g
Total Fat: 17g
Saturated Fat: 5g
Carbohydrates: 33g
Fiber: 2g
Sodium: 1933mg

This light, herby broth studded with carrots and golden chicken meatballs makes a satisfying meal on a crisp, early spring day— or, really, any day at all. If you'd like a more substantial soup, add cooked rice or gluten-free pasta to the broth just before serving.

FOR THE MEATBALLS
Oil for preparing the baking sheet
1 pound ground chicken
¾ cup cooked rice
½ cup chopped fresh basil
1½ ounces freshly grated Parmesan cheese, plus more for garnish
1 tablespoon Garlic Oil (page 202)
1 egg, lightly beaten
1¼ teaspoons salt
½ teaspoon freshly ground black pepper

FOR THE BROTH
1 tablespoon olive oil
1 tablespoon Garlic Oil (page 202)
1 large carrot, thinly sliced
5 cups homemade (onion- and garlic-free) chicken broth
4 cups baby spinach
½ cup chopped fresh basil

1. Preheat the oven to 400°F.

2. Line a large, rimmed baking sheet with parchment paper lightly coated with oil.

3. In a large bowl, combine the chicken, rice, basil, cheese, Garlic Oil, egg, salt, and pepper, and mix well. Form the mixture into 1-inch balls and arrange them on the prepared baking sheet. Bake in the preheated oven for about 25 minutes, until the meatballs are browned and cooked through. ▸

4. Meanwhile, make the broth. Heat the olive oil and Garlic Oil in a stockpot over medium-high heat. Add the carrots and cook, stirring, for 3 minutes, then add the broth and bring to a boil. Reduce the heat to low and simmer, uncovered, for about 10 minutes, until the carrots are tender. Stir in the spinach and basil, and cook just until wilted, for about 3 minutes.

5. To serve, place several meatballs in a serving bowl, and ladle the broth and vegetables over the top. Serve immediately, garnished with additional Parmesan cheese if desired.

Dijon-Roasted Pork Tenderloin

SERVES 8

PREP TIME: 5 MINUTES

COOK TIME: 60 MINUTES

Cooking Tip: For a juicy and tender pork roast, brine it overnight before cooking. In a large bowl or pot, combine 3 cups warm water, ¼ cup salt, and ¼ cup (packed) light brown sugar, and stir until the sugar and salt dissolve. Add 1 cup ice cubes and stir until the water is cold. Add the pork loin, making sure it is submerged. Cover and refrigerate for at least 12 hours (or up to 24). Drain the roast and pat it dry before proceeding with the recipe.

PER SERVING

Calories: 499
Protein: 65g
Total Fat: 22g
Saturated Fat: 8g
Carbohydrates: 5g
Fiber: 0g
Sodium: 604mg

There's nothing like roasted meat for Sunday dinner. This dish is simple to prepare and uses only a couple of common ingredients, but the end result is divine. Serve it with roasted vegetables and mashed potatoes for a satisfying and special meal.

1 pork loin roast (about 4 pounds), trimmed of excess fat
1 teaspoon salt
½ teaspoon pepper
¼ cup whole-grain Dijon mustard
¼ cup brown sugar

1. Preheat the oven to 425°F.

2. Season the roast all over with the salt and pepper, place it on a roasting rack in a roasting pan, and roast in the preheated oven for 30 minutes.

3. Brush the mustard over the entire roast, then sprinkle the brown sugar over it, pressing the sugar into the mustard.

4. Lower the oven heat to 375°F and continue roasting, basting now and then with the drippings, for about 30 minutes more, until a meat thermometer inserted into the center of the roast reads 145°F. Remove the roast from the oven, tent loosely with aluminum foil, and let rest for 10 minutes before slicing.

5. To serve, slice the roast into ½-inch-thick slices, and spoon a bit of the drippings over them.

Asian-Style Pork Meatballs

SERVES 4

PREP TIME: 10 MINUTES

COOK TIME: 40 MINUTES

Cooking Tip: Make smaller meatballs—1-inch instead of 2-inch—and serve them with tooth-picks for a simple, savory appetizer.

PER SERVING

Calories: 232
Protein: 38g
Total Fat: 5g
Saturated Fat: 2g
Carbohydrates: 7g
Fiber: 0g
Sodium: 1027mg

These spicy meatballs would make a great filling for a gluten-free sandwich roll (try a báhn mì-*style sandwich as on page 130), serve them atop Sesame Rice Noodles (page 117), or add them to a flavorful broth.*

Oil for preparing the baking sheet
1¼ pounds ground pork
¼ cup finely chopped fresh basil
1 tablespoon Garlic Oil (page 202)
2 scallions, green parts only, thinly sliced
1 tablespoon fish sauce
1 teaspoon onion- and garlic-free chili paste
1 tablespoon sugar
2 teaspoons cornstarch
1 teaspoon salt
1 teaspoon freshly ground black pepper

1. Preheat the oven to 350°F.

2. Line a large, rimmed baking sheet with lightly oiled parchment paper. In a large bowl, combine the pork, basil, Garlic Oil, scallions, fish sauce, chili paste, sugar, cornstarch, salt, and pepper, and mix to combine. With wet hands, form the mixture into 2-inch balls. Place the meatballs on the prepared baking sheet as they are formed.

3. Bake the meatballs in the preheated oven for about 40 minutes, until they are browned and cooked through. Serve hot.

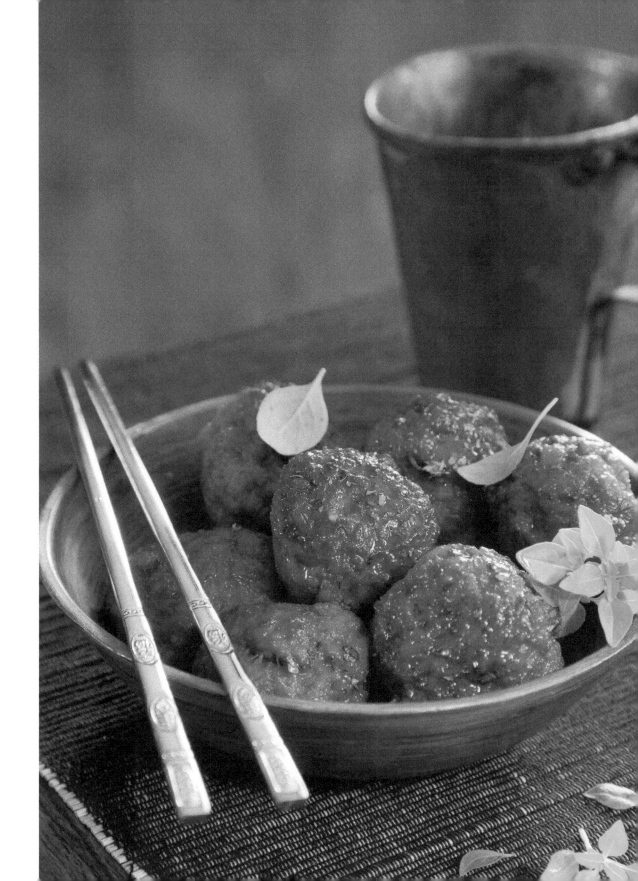

Chili-Rubbed Pork Chops with Raspberry Sauce

SERVES 4

PREP TIME: 5 MINUTES

COOK TIME: 10 MINUTES

Cooking Tip: For juicy pork chops, try quickly brining them before cooking. Combine 3 cups cold water, 3 tablespoons salt, and 3 tablespoons light-brown sugar in a large bowl, and stir until the sugar and salt dissolve. Add the pork chops, cover, and refrigerate for 30 minutes to 4 hours.

PER SERVING

Calories: 286
Protein: 35g
Total Fat: 14g
Saturated Fat: 3g
Carbohydrates: 7g
Fiber: 0g
Sodium: 657mg

Slightly spicy chili powder mingles with sweet raspberry preserves for a hot-sweet sensation that makes these chops irresistible. Serve them with grilled corn on the cob and sautéed chard or roasted broccoli for a special meal.

2 teaspoons gluten-free, onion- and garlic-free chili powder
½ teaspoon salt
1 teaspoon chopped fresh thyme
4 (6-ounce) bone-in, center-cut pork chops (about ½-inch thick)
2 tablespoons olive oil
¼ cup homemade (onion- and garlic-free) chicken broth
2 tablespoons seedless raspberry preserves

1. In a small bowl, combine the chili powder, salt, and thyme. Coat the pork chops all over with the spice mixture.

2. Heat the oil in a large skillet over medium-high heat. Cook the chops for about 3 minutes per side, until they are browned and cooked through. Transfer the cooked chops to a large plate or serving platter, tent loosely with foil, and keep warm.

3. Add the broth to the skillet and cook, stirring and scraping up any browned bits from the bottom of the pan, for about 30 seconds. Add the preserves and cook, stirring constantly, for 1 minute or until the sauce thickens.

4. Serve the pork chops brushed with the glaze.

Ginger-Sesame Grilled Flank Steak

SERVES 4

PREP TIME: 5 MINUTES, PLUS 30 MINUTES TO MARINATE

COOK TIME: 10 MINUTES

Cooking Tip: Marinating the steak overnight will infuse it with even more flavor. To do so, place the steak in the marinade and refrigerate for up to 24 hours. Bring the steak to room temperature by letting it sit on the countertop for about 20 minutes before cooking.

PER SERVING

Calories: 460
Protein: 48g
Total Fat: 25g
Saturated Fat: 8g
Carbohydrates: 9g
Fiber: 1g
Sodium: 1262mg

Flank steak is great for grilling, because it is extremely flavorful and very tender when cooked quickly over the high heat of a grill. Here it's infused with the kick of fresh ginger and the nuttiness of toasted sesame oil. Serve it with Coconut Rice (page 116) or Sesame Rice Noodles (page 117).

1 (5-inch) piece fresh ginger, minced
3 tablespoons dark sesame oil
2 tablespoons Garlic Oil (page 202)
2 teaspoons lime juice
1 tablespoon brown sugar
2 teaspoons salt
1 teaspoon pepper
1½ pounds flank steak
Oil for preparing the grill or grill pan

1. In large bowl or resealable plastic bag, combine the ginger, sesame oil, Garlic Oil, lime juice, brown sugar, salt, and pepper. Add the steak and turn to coat. Marinate the meat at room temperature for 30 minutes.

2. To cook the steak, oil a grill or grill pan, and heat to medium-high heat. Remove the steak from the marinade and cook on the grill for 4 to 5 minutes per side for medium-rare (cook a minute or two longer per side for medium, and even longer for well-done).

3. Tent the cooked steak loosely with aluminum foil and let rest for 10 minutes before slicing.

4. To serve, slice the steak across the grain into ⅛-inch-thick slices and serve immediately.

Grilled Carne Asada Tacos with Chimichurri Sauce

SERVES 4

PREP TIME: 10 MINUTES, PLUS 30 MINUTES TO MARINATE

COOK TIME: 10 MINUTES

Cooking Tip: Marinating the steak overnight will infuse it with even more flavor. To do so, place the steak in the marinade and refrigerate for up to 24 hours. Bring the steak to room temperature by letting it sit on the countertop for about 20 minutes before cooking.

PER SERVING

Calories: 559
Protein: 34g
Total Fat: 36g
Saturated Fat: 8g
Carbohydrates: 26g
Fiber: 4g
Sodium: 994mg

This quick-grilled steak makes the best filling for tacos. Here they're topped with Chimichurri Sauce (page 205), but they would be just as delicious topped with your favorite salsa and guacamole.

3 tablespoons olive oil, divided
2 tablespoons fresh lime juice, divided
1 teaspoon ground chipotle pepper
1 teaspoon salt
1 pound skirt steak
8 corn tortillas
Chimichurri Sauce (page 205)
¼ cup chopped fresh cilantro, for garnish

1. In a large bowl or resealable plastic bag, combine the olive oil, lime juice, ground chipotle, and salt. Add the steak and turn to coat. Marinate at room temperature for 30 minutes.

2. Heat a grill or grill pan to medium-high heat.

3. Grill the skirt steak to desired doneness, for 4 to 5 minutes per side for medium-rare. Remove the steak from the grill, tent it loosely with aluminum foil, and let rest for 10 minutes. Then slice it against the grain in ⅛-inch-thick slices.

4. Reduce the heat of the grill and set the tortillas on it to warm them, for about 1 minute.

5. Arrange 2 tortillas on each serving plate and top with several slices of the steak. Spoon the Chimichurri Sauce over the steak, garnish with cilantro, and serve immediately.

Quick Shepherd's Pie

SERVES 4

PREP TIME: 15 MINUTES

COOK TIME: 25 MINUTES

Substitution Tip: For a dairy-free version, replace the cream cheese and cream with ½ cup plus 2 tablespoons chicken broth. Also, in place of butter, use a dairy-free butter substitute. For a soy-free version, use the Low-FODMAP Worcestershire Sauce (page 203) or coconut aminos instead of the soy sauce.

PER SERVING

Calories: 692
Protein: 67g
Total Fat: 26g
Saturated Fat: 12g
Carbohydrates: 45g
Fiber: 7g
Sodium: 1780mg

Shepherd's pie is a wonderfully comforting dish consisting of ground meat and vegetables in hearty gravy, topped with a golden-brown layer of broiled mashed potatoes. This version is deceptively simple and quick to prepare. Just add a green salad or some steamed broccoli, and you have yourself a perfect Sunday-night meal. If desired, use ground lamb instead of beef for a more authentic flavor.

2 pounds potatoes, peeled and cubed

2 teaspoons salt, divided, plus additional if needed

2 tablespoons softened cream cheese

½ cup heavy cream

1 tablespoon olive oil

1¾ pounds ground beef or lamb

2 teaspoons freshly ground black pepper

1 carrot, diced

2 tablespoons butter

2 tablespoons gluten-free, low-FODMAP all-purpose flour (such as King Arthur's)

1 cup homemade (onion- and garlic-free) beef stock or broth

1 tablespoon Low-FODMAP Worcestershire Sauce (page 203) or gluten-free soy sauce

1 cup fresh or frozen green beans, cut into 1-inch pieces

1 tablespoon minced fresh thyme

1 tablespoon Garlic Oil (page 202)

2 tablespoons chopped fresh parsley, for garnish

1. Place the potatoes in a large saucepan and cover with water. Add 1 teaspoon of the salt and bring to a boil over high heat. Reduce the heat to medium, and simmer until the potatoes are tender, for about 12 minutes. ▶

Quick Shepherd's Pie *continued*

2. While the potatoes are cooking, heat the oil in a large skillet over medium-high heat. Add the meat, the remaining salt, and pepper. Cook, stirring and breaking up with a spatula, until the meat is browned, for about 4 minutes. Drain the excess fat from the pan. Add the carrot and cook, stirring occasionally, for another 5 minutes.

3. Drain the potatoes and transfer them to a large bowl. Add the cream cheese and cream, and mash with a potato masher until smooth. Taste and add more salt if needed.

4. In a small saucepan over medium heat, melt the butter. Add the flour and cook, whisking constantly, for 2 minutes. Whisk in the beef broth and Low-FODMAP Worcestershire Sauce or soy sauce, and cook until thickened, for about 1 more minute. Add the sauce to the meat mixture and stir in the green beans and thyme.

5. Preheat the broiler on high.

6. Transfer the meat mixture to a baking dish. Spoon the potato mixture over the top and spread out evenly. Broil for 3 to 4 minutes, until the potatoes are nicely browned. Remove from the oven and drizzle the Garlic Oil over the top. Serve hot, garnished with parsley.

Ginger-Orange Braised Short Ribs

SERVES 4

PREP TIME: 20 MINUTES

COOK TIME: 3 HOURS,
20 MINUTES

Substitution Tip: For a
soy-free version, substi-
tute coconut aminos for
the soy sauce.

PER SERVING

Calories: 577
Protein: 17g
Total Fat: 45g
Saturated Fat: 18g
Carbohydrates: 23g
Fiber: 0g
Sodium: 283mg

*A long braise in a spicy-sweet-salty mixture infuses these tender
short ribs with intense Asian flavor. After several hours in the oven,
the meat will fall from the bone. Serve this hearty dish over steamed
rice with a side of simple steamed vegetables.*

5 pounds beef short ribs, cut into 4-ounce pieces
1 cup gluten-free soy sauce
½ cup light-brown sugar
¼ cup rice vinegar
1 to 2 tablespoons onion- and garlic-free chili paste
1 tablespoon dark sesame oil
2 tablespoons minced fresh ginger
¾ teaspoon red-pepper flakes
4 tablespoons orange juice, divided
4 cups water
2 tablespoons lemon juice

1. Preheat the oven to 350°F.

2. Place the ribs, soy sauce, brown sugar, vinegar, chili paste,
sesame oil, ginger, red-pepper flakes, 2 tablespoons of the orange
juice, and water in a large Dutch oven. Cover the pot and cook in
the preheated oven for 3 hours, until the meat is very tender and
falling apart. Take the pot out of the oven and carefully transfer
the ribs to a plate. Set aside.

3. Raise the oven temperature to 425°F.

4. Skim the fat off the top of the cooking liquid. Bring the liquid to a
boil over medium-high heat, and cook until it is reduced to about
1¼ cups, for about 10 minutes. Strain the liquid through a fine-meshed
sieve and discard the solids. Return the liquid to the pot and stir in the
remaining 2 tablespoons of the orange juice and the lemon juice.

5. Return the ribs to the pot in the oven. Cook for about
10 minutes, until the liquid becomes a thick glaze. Serve hot.

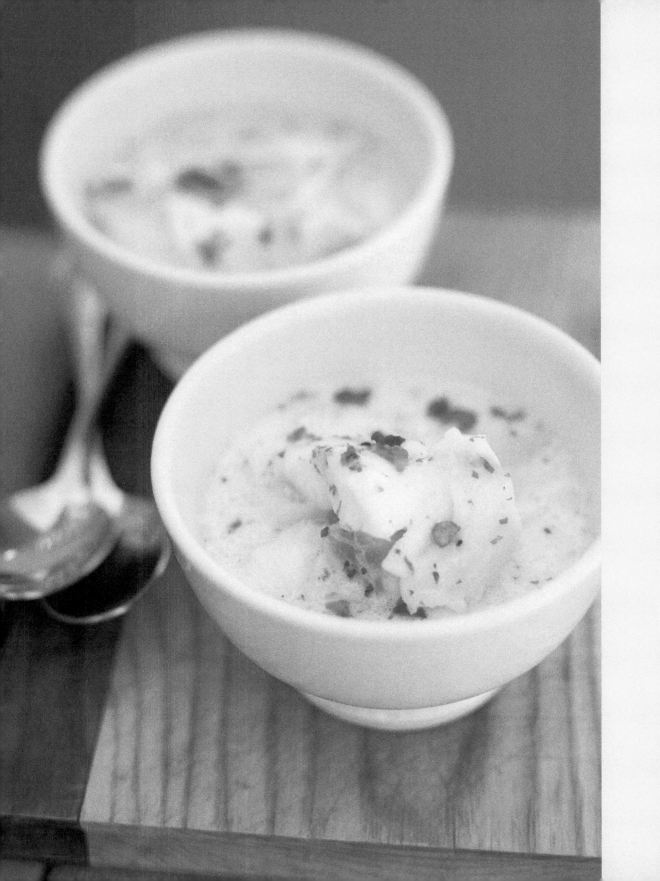

9

Fish and Seafood

Classic Fish Chowder

SERVES 4

PREP TIME: 10 MINUTES

COOK TIME: 40 MINUTES

Tip: To make this allergen-free, omit the heavy cream and replace it with unsweetened coconut milk.

PER SERVING

Calories: 662
Protein: 73g
Total Fat: 14g
Saturated Fat: 5g
Carbohydrates: 50g
Fiber: 6g
Sodium: 1902mg

This hearty fish chowder is flavored with leeks (using just the low-FODMAP, green part), salt pork, and fresh thyme. If you have fish stock on hand, use it instead of vegetable broth for an even more authentic fish chowder. Cod is a great fish for chowder because it is meaty and firm enough to hold its shape after cooking in the broth, but you can substitute any firm whitefish you like, such as haddock, halibut, or snapper.

4 slices bacon, cut into ¼-inch dices
6 green onions (green part only), thinly sliced
1 yellow bell pepper, seeded and chopped
6 cups homemade (onion- and garlic-free) vegetable broth
2 pounds red potatoes, cubed (unpeeled)
1 zucchini, cut into cubes (unpeeled)
1 teaspoon salt
½ teaspoon freshly ground black pepper
3 pounds skinless cod fillets, preferably over 1-inch thick, pinbones removed, cut into chunks
1 tablespoon chopped fresh thyme
½ cup heavy cream

1. Heat a stockpot over low heat. Add the bacon and cook until it is crispy. Raise the heat to medium and cook until the pork is golden brown and crisp. Using a slotted spoon, remove the pork from the pot and reserve.

2. Add the green onions and bell pepper to the fat in the stockpot. Cook, stirring occasionally, for about 8 minutes, until the peppers are soft.

3. Stir in the broth, potatoes, zucchini, salt, and pepper. Add a little water if needed to cover the potatoes with liquid. Raise the heat to high and bring to a boil. Cover and cook until the potatoes are tender, about 10 minutes. Mash a few of the potato slices with the back of a wooden spoon to thicken the broth a bit.

4. Reduce the heat to low. Add the fish and fresh thyme and cook for about 5 minutes, until the fish is almost cooked through. Remove from the heat and let the chowder sit for about 10 minutes.

5. Stir in the coconut milk and warm over low heat just until heated through. Serve hot, garnished with the reserved bacon.

Crunchy Homemade Fish Sticks

SERVES 4

PREP TIME: 10 MINUTES

COOK TIME: 15 MINUTES

Substitution Tip: For a dairy-free version, swap out the lactose-free milk for rice milk or coconut milk.

PER SERVING

Calories: 310
Protein: 34g
Total Fat: 4g
Saturated Fat: 1g
Carbohydrates: 33g
Fiber: 1g
Sodium: 842mg

Sometimes fish sticks really hit the spot. These are coated in crunchy cornflake crumbs, so they're gluten-free but still nice and crisp. Serve with your favorite veggies and a bit of Low-FODMAP Spicy Ketchup (page 219).

3½ cups gluten-free cornflakes
⅓ cup rice flour
1 egg
2 tablespoons lactose-free milk
1 pound firm whitefish fillets, such as snapper, skin removed, cut into 1-by-3-inch pieces
1 teaspoon salt
Cooking spray

1. Preheat the oven to 400°F.

2. Line a large, rimmed baking sheet with parchment paper.

3. In a food processor, pulse the cornflakes to make fine crumbs, and place the crumbs in a wide, shallow bowl. Next, place the rice flour in another wide, shallow bowl. In a separate wide, shallow bowl, beat together the egg and milk.

4. Season the fish all over with salt and dredge each piece in the flour. Next, dip each piece of fish in the egg mixture and then into the cornflake crumbs. Arrange the fish pieces on the prepared baking sheet. Spray the fish lightly with cooking spray and bake in the preheated oven for about 15 minutes, until golden brown and crisp. Serve hot.

Pecan-Crusted Maple-Mustard Salmon

SERVES 4

PREP TIME: 5 MINUTES

COOK TIME: 12 MINUTES

Substitution Tip: For a nut-free version, you can substitute gluten-free bread crumbs for the pecans.

PER SERVING

Calories: 305
Protein: 34g
Total Fat: 16g
Saturated Fat: 2g
Carbohydrates: 8g
Fiber: 1g
Sodium: 165mg

Spicy mustard, sweet maple syrup, and crunchy pecans make an appetizing crust for salmon fillets. Serve this dish with Green Beans and New Potatoes with Tomato (page 111) or Rice Pilaf with Vegetables (page 115).

Cooking spray
2 tablespoons Dijon mustard
2 tablespoons maple syrup
4 (6-ounce) salmon fillets
½ cup finely chopped pecans

1. Preheat the oven to 425°F.

2. Coat a baking dish with cooking spray. In a small bowl, stir together the mustard and maple syrup. Arrange the salmon fillets in a single layer in the baking dish. Spread the mustard–maple syrup mixture over the tops of the fillets. Sprinkle the pecans on top, pressing them into the mustard mixture.

3. Bake in the preheated oven for about 12 minutes, until the salmon is cooked through and flakes easily with a fork. Serve immediately.

Thai Sweet Chili Broiled Salmon

SERVES 4

PREP TIME: 5 MINUTES,
PLUS 30 MINUTES TO
MARINATE

COOK TIME: 10 MINUTES

Substitution Tip: For a
soy-free version, you can
substitute either fish
sauce or coconut aminos
for the gluten-free
soy sauce.

PER SERVING

Calories: 291
Protein: 34g
Total Fat: 11g
Saturated Fat: 2g
Carbohydrates: 13g
Fiber: 1g
Sodium: 812mg

If you've got a batch of Thai Sweet Chili Sauce (page 210) on hand, this recipe is seriously quick and easy to prepare. Even if you make the sauce from scratch, you can have this spicy-sweet salmon on the table with less than 20 minutes of active prep. Serve with steamed broccoli and white rice.

6 tablespoons homemade Thai Sweet Chili Sauce (page 210)
3 tablespoons gluten-free soy sauce
1 tablespoon finely grated fresh ginger
4 (6-ounce) salmon fillets
2 scallions (green part only), thinly sliced
1 tablespoon chopped fresh cilantro
1½ teaspoons toasted sesame seeds

1. In a large bowl, combine the chili sauce, soy sauce, and ginger, and mix well. Add the fish, turning until evenly coated. Cover the bowl and marinate fish in the refrigerator for 30 minutes.

2. To cook the fish, heat the broiler to high and line a rimmed baking sheet with foil.

3. Arrange the salmon fillets skin-side down on the prepared baking sheet. Brush some of the marinade over the fish, coating generously. Broil for about 8 to 10 minutes, until just cooked through. Serve immediately, garnished with scallions, cilantro, and sesame seeds.

Red Snapper with Creole Sauce

SERVES 4

PREP TIME: 10 MINUTES

COOK TIME: 20 MINUTES

Cooking Tip: To get this dish on the table even quicker, season the fish with salt and pepper, and bake it in a 400°F oven for about 8 minutes while you make the sauce.

PER SERVING

Calories: 281
Protein: 46g
Total Fat: 7g
Saturated Fat: 1g
Carbohydrates: 7g
Fiber: 2g
Sodium: 588mg

Creole sauce is quick to make; you can easily get this dinner on the table in less than 30 minutes. And it's great for dressing up shrimp, chicken, or, as suggested here, red snapper fillets. Serve this dish with steamed rice and a crisp green salad.

1 tablespoon olive oil
1 tablespoon Garlic Oil (page 202)
½ medium green bell pepper, diced
1 (14½-ounce) can onion- and garlic-free diced tomatoes with juice
2 scallions (green part only), thinly sliced
1 tablespoon red-wine vinegar
1 teaspoon gluten-free soy sauce or coconut aminos
½ teaspoon dried basil
½ teaspoon salt
½ teaspoon freshly ground black pepper
Dash of hot-pepper sauce
4 (6-ounce) red-snapper fillets
¼ cup chopped fresh basil

1. Heat the olive oil and Garlic Oil in a large skillet over medium-high heat. Add the bell pepper and cook, stirring, until softened, for about 5 minutes. Add the tomatoes with their juice, scallions, vinegar, soy sauce, basil, salt, pepper, and hot sauce and bring to a boil.

2. Reduce the heat to low, add the fish, and spoon the saucy tomato mixture over the top. Cover the pan and cook until the fish is cooked through and flakes easily with a fork, for about 10 minutes. Serve immediately, with sauce spooned over the top and garnished with basil.

Spicy Salmon Burgers with Cilantro-Lime Mayo

SERVES 4

PREP TIME: 10 MINUTES

COOK TIME: 5 MINUTES

Cooking Tip: If you don't have a grill or grill pan, simply cook these patties in a bit of olive oil in a large skillet. Heat the oil in the skillet over medium-high heat, then cook the patties for about 2 minutes per side, until browned and cooked through.

PER SERVING

Calories: 455
Protein: 29g
Total Fat: 19g
Saturated Fat: 3g
Carbohydrates: 48g
Fiber: 6g
Sodium: 841mg

Lighter than a traditional beef burger but no less flavorful, these spicy patties make a crowd-pleasing filler for your burger buns. Serve them at your next barbecue or for a light supper on a warm summer evening. Classic Coleslaw (page 106) would make a fine accompaniment.

FOR THE MAYO
¼ cup mayonnaise
1 tablespoon chopped fresh cilantro
Zest and juice of 1 lime
⅛ teaspoon salt
⅛ teaspoon freshly ground black pepper

FOR THE BURGERS
1 pound salmon fillet, skinned and cut into pieces
¼ cup gluten-free plain bread crumbs
2 tablespoons chopped fresh cilantro
1 small jalapeño chile, seeded and diced
2 tablespoons lime juice
½ teaspoon salt
¼ teaspoon freshly ground black pepper
Cooking spray

TO SERVE
4 gluten-free hamburger buns, toasted
½ medium cucumber, thinly sliced
1 large tomato, sliced
4 lettuce leaves

1. To make the mayo, combine the mayonnaise, cilantro, lime zest and juice, and salt and pepper in a small bowl, and stir to mix well. Cover and refrigerate until ready to use. ▶

Spicy Salmon Burgers
with Cilantro-Lime Mayo *continued*

2. To make the burgers, pulse the salmon in a food processor until coarsely chopped. Add the bread crumbs, cilantro, jalapeño, lime juice, salt, and pepper, and pulse until well combined. Form the mixture into 4 (¾-inch-thick) patties.

3. Coat a grill or grill pan with cooking spray and heat over medium-high heat. Cook the salmon burgers for about 2 minutes per side, until browned and cooked through.

4. To serve, spread some of the cilantro-lime mayo onto the bottom half of each burger bun. Top with a salmon patty, a few slices of cucumber, a tomato slice, a lettuce leaf, and the top half of the bun. Serve immediately.

Grilled Halibut Tacos with Cabbage Slaw

SERVES 4

PREP TIME: 10 MINUTES, PLUS 20 MINUTES FOR REFRIGERATION

COOK TIME: 10 MINUTES

Cooking Tip: If cooking the fish on a grill, use a grilling basket so you don't end up losing half of your fish in the fire when you attempt to flip it over.

PER SERVING

Calories: 547
Protein: 36g
Total Fat: 25g
Saturated Fat: 4g
Carbohydrates: 47g
Fiber: 9g
Sodium: 983mg

In this taco recipe, the fish is grilled instead of fried, making this a lighter version of the classic dish. The chili spice rub and smokiness from the grill make up for any flavor lost from skipping the deep fryer.

FOR THE FISH TACOS
4 teaspoons gluten-, onion-, and garlic-free chili powder
2 tablespoons lime juice
2 tablespoons olive oil
1 teaspoon ground cumin
1 teaspoon salt
½ teaspoon freshly ground black pepper
4 (6-ounce) halibut fillets
Cooking spray
12 corn tortillas, warmed
½ avocado, thinly sliced

FOR THE SLAW
½ cup mayonnaise
2 tablespoons chopped fresh cilantro
Zest and juice of 1 lime
1 teaspoon sugar
⅛ teaspoon salt
⅛ teaspoon pepper
3 cups finely shredded green cabbage

1. In a small bowl, combine the chili powder, lime juice, oil, cumin, salt, and pepper. Rub the spice mixture all over the fish fillets and refrigerate for about 20 minutes. ▶

2. While the fish is marinating, make the coleslaw. In a large bowl, combine the mayonnaise, cilantro, lime zest and juice, sugar, salt, and pepper, and stir to mix. Add the cabbage and toss well. Cover and refrigerate until ready to serve.

3. To cook the fish, spray a grill or grill pan with cooking spray and heat it to medium-high.

4. Cook the fish for 3 to 5 minutes per side, until it flakes easily with a fork. Transfer to a cutting board and break into chunks.

5. To serve, place 2 tortillas on each serving plate. Top with some of the fish and a handful of coleslaw.

Fish with Thai Red Curry Sauce

SERVES 4

PREP TIME: 10 MINUTES

COOK TIME: 30 MINUTES

Cooking Tip: Kaffir lime leaves are available in Asian groceries and in the international foods section of many super-markets. If you can't find them where you live, you can order them online. They freeze well, so stock up and have them on hand whenever you need them.

Calories: 571
Protein: 23g
Total Fat: 35g
Saturated Fat: 7g
Carbohydrates: 44g
Fiber: 5g
Sodium: 2261mg

Living the low-FODMAP lifestyle, unfortunately, means giving up on restaurant curries, but that doesn't mean you can't still enjoy dishes like this at home. This Thai-style curry has a coconut milk–based sauce that is loaded with flavor from homemade low-FODMAP Thai Red Curry Paste (page 209). Serve it over steamed white rice.

1 tablespoon grapeseed oil
¼ cup Thai Red Curry Paste (page 209)
2½ cups coconut milk
2 tablespoons fish sauce
2 Kaffir lime leaves
1 sweet potato, peeled and diced
1 zucchini, diced
1 cup green beans, cut into 1-inch pieces
1½ pounds fish fillet
¼ cup crushed toasted peanuts
¼ cup chopped fresh cilantro

1. Heat the oil in a large saucepan over medium-high heat. Add the curry paste and cook, stirring, for about 1 minute. Stir in the coconut milk, fish sauce, and lime leaves, and bring to a boil.

2. Add the sweet potato, reduce the heat to low, and simmer for 10 minutes. Stir in the zucchini and green beans, and continue to cook for about 10 minutes more, until the vegetables are tender.

3. Add the fish and cook for 7 to 9 minutes more, until the fish is cooked through. Serve hot, garnished with peanuts and cilantro.

Red Snapper with Sweet Potato Crust and Cilantro-Lime Sauce

SERVES 4

PREP TIME: 15 MINUTES

COOK TIME: 15 MINUTES

Substitution Tip: For a dairy-free version, use a vegan butter substitute in place of the butter.

PER SERVING

Calories: 653
Protein: 49g
Total Fat: 39g
Saturated Fat: 8g
Carbohydrates: 26g
Fiber: 4g
Sodium: 1357mg

Shredded sweet potatoes form a sweet, crispy crust for flaky snapper and also prevent the fish from drying out during cooking. A tangy cilantro-lime sauce balances the sweetness of the potatoes while adding bright-green color to the dish. Serve the fish atop mixed greens for a complete meal.

FOR THE SAUCE
1 cup chopped fresh cilantro
Juice of 2 limes
½ cup olive oil
1 tablespoon Garlic Oil (page 202)
1 teaspoon salt
½ teaspoon freshly ground black pepper
½ teaspoon sugar

FOR THE FISH
½ cup gluten-free all-purpose flour
1 egg plus 2 egg whites
4 (6-ounce) snapper fillets
1 teaspoon salt
½ teaspoon freshly ground black pepper
1 tablespoon grapeseed oil
2 tablespoons butter
2 sweet potatoes, peeled and shredded

1. To make the sauce, combine the cilantro, lime juice, olive oil, Garlic Oil, salt, pepper, and sugar in a blender or food processor and process until smooth.

2. Preheat the oven to 375°F. Place the flour in a wide, shallow bowl. Beat together the egg and egg whites in a second wide, shallow bowl. Season the fish on both sides with salt and pepper.

3. To prepare the fish, heat the oil and butter in a large, oven-safe skillet over medium-high heat. Place a handful of sweet potatoes in the skillet, making a bed roughly the size and shape of each fish fillet. Dredge the fish fillets in the flour, then the egg, and set on top of the sweet potatoes. Cook until the sweet potatoes are crisp and golden brown, for about 4 minutes. Using a spatula, lift the crusted fish out of the pan, and use your other hand to create another bed of sweet potatoes. Flip the fish over onto the new sweet potato bed. Repeat with the other pieces of fish. Place the skillet in the preheated oven and cook for 5 to 7 minutes more, until the bottom crust is crisp and golden brown and the fish is cooked through.

4. Serve hot, with the sauce drizzled over the top.

Roasted Garlic Shrimp and Red Peppers

SERVES 4

PREP TIME: 5 MINUTES

COOK TIME: 17 MINUTES

Substitution Tip: For a shellfish-free version, use a firm whitefish, like cod or halibut, in place of the shrimp. Cut the fish fillets into 1-by-3-inch strips and proceed with the recipe as written.

PER SERVING

Calories: 260
Protein: 50g
Total Fat: 4g
Saturated Fat: 0g
Carbohydrates: 9g
Fiber: 3g
Sodium: 1099mg

Using Garlic Oil (page 202) in place of fresh garlic gives these plump, juicy prawns and peppers plenty of garlic flavor without the FODMAPs. Serve over creamy polenta along with a crisp green salad.

2 pounds peeled and deveined shrimp (tails left intact)
2 red bell peppers, cut into 1½-inch triangles
4 tablespoons Garlic Oil (page 202)
1½ tablespoons smoked paprika
¾ teaspoon cayenne
1 teaspoon salt
½ teaspoon freshly ground black pepper
1 tablespoon chopped fresh oregano

1. Preheat the oven to 400°F.

2. In a large baking dish, combine the shrimp, peppers, Garlic Oil, paprika, cayenne, salt, and pepper, and toss to coat. Spread the shrimp and peppers out in a single layer.

3. Roast the shrimp and peppers in the preheated oven for 10 minutes. Using tongs, flip the shrimp and peppers over, sprinkle the oregano over the top, and continue to roast for another 5 to 7 minutes, until the shrimp are cooked through. Serve hot.

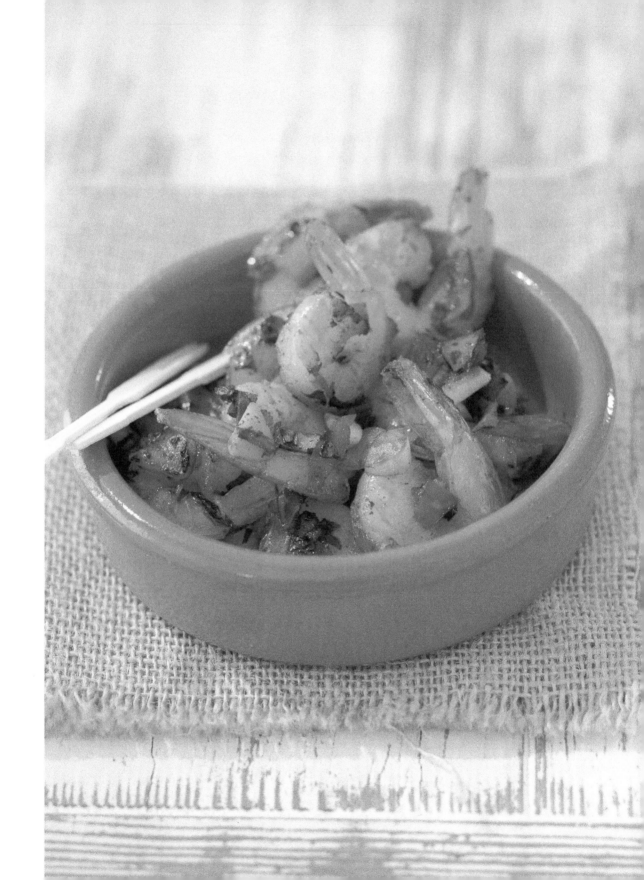

Risotto with Smoked Salmon and Dill

SERVES 4

PREP TIME: 5 MINUTES

COOK TIME: 30 MINUTES

Substitution Tip: For a dairy-free version, omit the Parmesan cheese and substitute ½ cup nutritional yeast, plus additional for garnish.

PER SERVING

Calories: 634
Protein: 37g
Total Fat: 23g
Saturated Fat: 13g
Carbohydrates: 64g
Fiber: 2g
Sodium: 3329mg

Creamy and satisfying risotto makes a great, comforting meal and is especially appreciated when you can't have pasta. This version only uses a handful of ingredients, but the end result is extra special, because several of them—leeks, smoked salmon, Parmesan cheese, and fresh dill—pack loads of flavor. Serve it with a crisp green salad with a lemony dressing for an easy and filling meal.

6 cups homemade (onion- and garlic-free) vegetable broth
3 tablespoons butter
1 medium leek (green part only), halved lengthwise and thinly sliced
1½ cups Arborio rice
½ cup dry white wine
1 teaspoon salt
1 tablespoon minced fresh dill
¾ cup freshly grated Parmesan cheese, divided
8 ounces smoked salmon

1. In a large saucepan, heat the broth to a simmer over medium-high heat. Reduce the heat to low and keep warm.

2. In a stockpot or Dutch oven, melt the butter over medium-high heat. Add the leek and cook, stirring, until softened, for about 5 minutes. Add the rice and cook, stirring, for about 2 minutes, until all of the grains of rice are well coated in butter. Add the wine and cook, stirring and scraping up any browned bits on the bottom of the pan, until the liquid has been absorbed. Add the salt and a ladleful of stock.

3. Cook, stirring, until the liquid has mostly evaporated. Continue to add broth a ladleful at a time and cook, stirring frequently, after each addition until most of the liquid has been absorbed. Cook for about 25 minutes total, until all of the broth has been used up and the rice is tender.

4. Stir in the dill and ½ cup of the cheese. Just before serving, stir in the salmon. Serve hot, garnished with the remaining cheese.

Moroccan Fish Stew with Cod, Fennel, Potatoes, and Tomatoes

SERVES 4

PREP TIME: 5 MINUTES

COOK TIME: 15 MINUTES

Substitution Tip: If cod isn't available, you can substitute any firm whitefish, such as halibut, snapper, or mahi-mahi.

PER SERVING

Calories: 306
Protein: 28g
Total Fat: 6g
Saturated Fat: 1g
Carbohydrates: 33g
Fiber: 5g
Sodium: 636mg

This bright stew is both light and satisfyingly filling. Serve it with a crisp green salad and crusty, gluten-free rolls for sopping up the delicious broth.

1 tablespoon olive oil
1 tablespoon minced fresh ginger
1 teaspoon ground cumin
1 teaspoon ground turmeric
1 cinnamon stick
⅛ teaspoon cayenne
1 (14½-ounce) can onion- and garlic-free diced tomatoes with juice
1 large fennel bulb, cored and thinly sliced
1 pound new potatoes, halved or quartered
1 cup water
1 teaspoon salt
½ teaspoon freshly ground black pepper
1¼ pounds cod fillets, cut into 2-inch chunks
2 tablespoons Garlic Oil (page 202)
2 tablespoons chopped fresh parsley

1. Heat the olive oil in a large skillet over medium heat.

2. Add the ginger, cumin, turmeric, cinnamon stick, and cayenne and cook, stirring, for 1 minute. Stir in the tomatoes with their juice, fennel, potatoes, water, salt, and pepper. Cook, stirring frequently, for about 10 minutes, until the potatoes are tender.

3. Add the fish and cook until the fish is cooked through, for about 5 minutes. Remove and discard the cinnamon stick.

4. Serve hot, garnished with a drizzle of Garlic Oil and a sprinkling of parsley.

Fish and Potato Pie

1

SERVES 6

PREP TIME: 15 MINUTES

COOK TIME: 50 MINUTES

Substitution Tip:
For a dairy-free version,
substitute olive oil
for the butter and omit
the cheese.

PER SERVING

Calories: 366
Protein: 34g
Total Fat: 16g
Saturated Fat: 10g
Carbohydrates: 22g
Fiber: 4g
Sodium: 1312mg

Fish pie is simple, filling, and—if properly prepared—good for you. This lighter-than-usual version is topped with mashed potatoes and combines smoked and fresh fish. All you need to round out this meal is to add a crisp green salad.

2 large potatoes
4 tablespoons butter, divided
1½ teaspoons salt, divided
1 teaspoon freshly ground black pepper, divided
¾ pound smoked whitefish (such as haddock),
  cut into bite-size pieces
¾ pound skinless salmon fillet, cut into ½-inch pieces
1 medium carrot, coarsely grated
2 (8-inch) stalks celery, coarsely grated
4 cups chopped fresh spinach
4 ounces grated sharp white cheddar cheese

1. Preheat the oven to 400°F.

2. Bring a pot of salted water to a boil. Add the potatoes and cook for 10 to 12 minutes, until the potatoes are tender. Drain and then mash the potatoes along with 2 tablespoons of the butter, ¾ teaspoon of the salt, and ½ teaspoon of the pepper.

3. In a large baking dish, toss together the smoked fish, salmon, carrot, celery, and spinach. Season with the remaining ¾ teaspoon salt and ½ teaspoon pepper. Spread the mixture out in an even layer. Spread the mashed potatoes over the top in an even layer. Melt the remaining 2 tablespoons of butter and drizzle it over the top. Sprinkle the cheese over the top.

4. Bake in the preheated oven for 30 to 40 minutes, until the top is golden brown and the dish is hot all the way through. Serve immediately.

Indian-Spiced Prawns with Coconut Milk

SERVES 4

PREP TIME: 10 MINUTES

COOK TIME: 10 MINUTES

Substitution Tip: For a shellfish-free version, omit the prawns and substitute a firm white-fish, such as halibut or snapper. Cut the fish fillets into 1-by-3-inch strips before adding to the pan, and proceed with the recipe as written.

PER SERVING

Calories: 305
Protein: 38g
Total Fat: 17g
Saturated Fat: 10g
Carbohydrates: 4g
Fiber: 2g
Sodium: 392mg

Creamy coconut milk makes a delicious brothy base for this spicy prawn dish. Serve it over steamed white or brown rice, which will soak up the sauce. To make this a complete meal, just add a green salad or some steamed or roasted vegetables.

2 red jalapeño or serrano chiles, seeded and chopped
1-inch piece peeled fresh ginger, sliced
1 tablespoon grapeseed oil
1 teaspoon black mustard seeds
½ teaspoon fenugreek seeds
½ teaspoon ground turmeric
½ teaspoon cracked black peppercorns
1½ pounds peeled and deveined prawns
¾ cup canned coconut milk
½ cup chopped fresh basil
Juice of 1 lime
2 tablespoons chopped fresh cilantro

1. In a food processor, pulse the chiles and ginger with 3 tablespoons of water until finely chopped.

2. Heat the oil in a heavy skillet over medium-high heat and add the mustard and fenugreek seeds. Cook, shaking the pan, for about 10 seconds. Add the chile-ginger purée and reduce the heat to low. Cook, stirring, for about 3 minutes.

3. Stir in the turmeric, peppercorns, prawns, and coconut milk, and bring to a simmer. Cook for 2 to 3 minutes, until the prawns are cooked through and fully opaque. Stir in the basil and lime juice, and serve immediately, garnished with cilantro.

Steamed Mussels with Saffron-Infused Cream

SERVES 4

PREP TIME: 5 MINUTES

COOK TIME: 15 MINUTES

Substitution Tip: For a shellfish-free version, substitute a firm, meaty fish—cod, halibut, or even salmon would be lovely—for the mussels. Cut the fish into 2-inch chunks and add it along with the cream and pepper. Cover the pot and cook just until the fish is cooked through, for 3 to 5 minutes.

PER SERVING

Calories: 599
Protein: 55g
Total Fat: 26g
Saturated Fat: 8g
Carbohydrates: 24g
Fiber: 2g
Sodium: 1779mg

Affordable, widely available, easy to cook, and delicious, mussels are an underappreciated shellfish. Here they're steamed in a saffron-infused, wine-based broth. Serve them in bowls with a ladleful of the scrumptious broth and slices of crusty, gluten-free baguette to sop up the tasty juices.

2 tablespoons olive oil
1 tablespoon Garlic Oil (page 202)
1 large bulb fennel, thinly sliced
1 cup dry white wine
Large pinch saffron threads
¾ teaspoon salt
¾ cup heavy cream
¼ teaspoon freshly ground pepper
4 pounds cultivated mussels, rinsed well
2 tablespoons chopped fresh flat-leaf parsley

1. Heat the olive oil and Garlic Oil in a stockpot over medium heat.

2. Add the fennel and cook, stirring frequently, until softened, for about 5 minutes. Add the wine, saffron, and salt, and bring to a boil. Stir in the cream, pepper, and mussels.

3. Cover the pot and cook for about 6 minutes or until all of the mussels have opened (discard any mussels that don't open after 8 minutes of cooking). Serve the mussels and broth in bowls, garnished with the parsley.

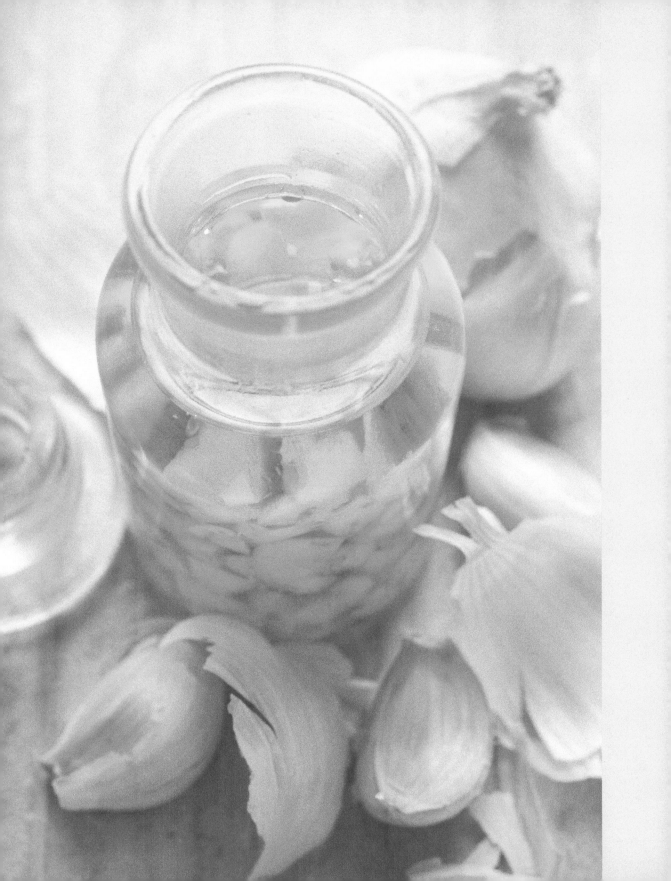

10

Sauces, Dressings, and Condiments

Garlic Oil

MAKES ABOUT 1 CUP

PREP TIME: 5 MINUTES

COOK TIME: 5 MINUTES

Cooking Tip: The same trick works using onion. Replace the garlic with ½ onion, thinly sliced, or use a combination of onion and garlic (¼ onion and 3 cloves of garlic).

PER SERVING

(1 TABLESPOON)

Calories: 108
Protein: 0g
Total Fat: 13g
Saturated Fat: 2g
Carbohydrates: 0g
Fiber: 0g
Sodium: 0mg

Garlic is off limits on the low-FODMAP diet, but this garlic-infused oil—made by steeping fresh garlic in olive oil and then straining out the FODMAP-containing solids—allows you to enjoy the garlic flavor essential to so many recipes. Keep a jar on hand, and you're guaranteed to find a million uses for it.

1 cup olive oil
6 cloves garlic, sliced

1. Heat the olive oil in a small saucepan over medium-low heat.

2. Add the garlic and cook at a low simmer, stirring often, for 5 minutes.

3. Strain the oil through a fine-meshed sieve and discard the solids.

4. Refrigerate the oil in a covered container for up to a week.

Low-FODMAP Worcestershire Sauce

MAKES ABOUT 1½ CUPS

PREP TIME: 5 MINUTES

COOK TIME: 20 MINUTES

Substitution Tip: For a soy-free version, substitute coconut aminos for the gluten-free soy sauce.

(1 TABLESPOON)

Calories: 21
Protein: 0g
Total Fat: 0g
Saturated Fat: 0g
Carbohydrates: 2g
Fiber: 0g
Sodium: 17mg

Cooking low-FODMAP foods can be frustrating, as even the most innocent-seeming recipes often contain hidden FODMAPs. Store-bought Worcestershire sauce, for example, contains both onions and garlic. This version omits them, using other flavorful ingredients like balsamic vinegar, ginger, cumin and fennel seeds, and cinnamon to make up for lost flavor. Use this condiment as a substitute in any recipe that calls for Worcestershire sauce.

2 cups rice vinegar
1 teaspoon balsamic vinegar
½ cup gluten-free soy sauce or tamari
¼ cup light-brown sugar
1 teaspoon ground ginger
1 teaspoon dry mustard
1 teaspoon cumin seeds
½ teaspoon fennel seeds
½ teaspoon ground cinnamon
½ teaspoon freshly ground black pepper

1. In a medium saucepan, combine all of the ingredients and bring to a boil over medium-high heat. Reduce the heat to low and simmer, stirring occasionally, for 20 minutes or until the liquid has been reduced by about half.

2. Strain the mixture through a fine-meshed sieve, discarding the solids, and let cool to room temperature. Store in a covered container in the refrigerator for up to 3 months.

Homemade Mayonnaise

MAKES ABOUT ¾ CUP

PREP TIME: 5 MINUTES

COOK TIME: NONE

Substitution Tip: For an egg-free version, replace the egg yolk with 2 teaspoons ground flaxseed stirred into 2 tablespoons hot water and cooled to room temperature.

PER SERVING

(1 TABLESPOON)

Calories: 113
Protein: 0g
Total Fat: 13g
Saturated Fat: 2g
Carbohydrates: 0g
Fiber: 0g
Sodium: 99mg

Once you've tried homemade mayonnaise, you just might swear off the store-bought kind for good. It's easy to make and tastes so much better than the jarred stuff that there's just no comparison. This classic version uses egg yolk and olive oil flavored with lemon juice, vinegar, Dijon mustard, and salt. Use a yolk from a pasteurized egg to avoid potential food poisoning.

1 large pasteurized egg yolk
1½ teaspoons fresh lemon juice
1 teaspoon white wine vinegar
¼ teaspoon Dijon mustard
½ teaspoon salt
¾ cup light olive oil

1. In a blender or food processor, combine the egg yolk, lemon juice, vinegar, mustard, and salt, and process to combine. With the processor running, slowly add the oil. Continue processing until all of the oil has been added and the mixture is thick.

2. Transfer to a storage container and store, covered, in the refrigerator for up to 3 days.

Chimichurri Sauce

MAKES ABOUT 1½ CUPS

PREP TIME: 5 MINUTES

COOK TIME: NONE

Cooking Tip: For a different texture—or if you simply don't have access to a blender or food processor—make the sauce by finely chopping the herbs by hand and stirring them together with the oils, lemon juice, and spices.

PER SERVING

(¼ CUP)

Calories: 88
Protein: 1g
Total Fat: 9g
Saturated Fat: 1g
Carbohydrates: 3g
Fiber: 1g
Sodium: 203mg

Garlicky and bright, chimichurri is a popular condiment in many Latin American cuisines. Made with lemon juice and lots of fresh herbs—usually parsley and cilantro—it adds a flavorful and fresh finishing touch to many dishes. Use it to top grilled steak, chicken, fish, prawns, vegetables, tofu, or eggs, or stir it into a stew for added flavor.

1 cup fresh flat-leaf parsley
¼ cup lemon juice
¼ cup olive oil
¼ cup Garlic Oil (page 202)
¼ cup fresh cilantro
¾ teaspoon red-pepper flakes
½ teaspoon ground cumin
½ teaspoon salt

1. Combine all the ingredients in a blender or food processor and process until smooth.

2. Use immediately or cover and refrigerate for up to a week.

Cilantro-Coconut Pesto

MAKES ABOUT 1 CUP

PREP TIME: 5 MINUTES

COOK TIME: NONE

Substitution Tip: The peanuts add texture and a nice nutty flavor, but they are optional. For a nut-free version, omit the peanuts or substitute pumpkin seeds (pepitas) or sunflower seeds.

PER SERVING

(2 TABLESPOONS)

Calories: 90
Protein: 2g
Total Fat: 8g
Saturated Fat: 3g
Carbohydrates: 3g
Fiber: 1g
Sodium: 23mg

This unusual pesto substitutes cilantro for the more typical basil. Combined with coconut and peanuts, the result is a South or Southeast Asian flavor. Use it as a spread for gluten-free bread or crackers, toss it with cooked rice noodles, or dollop it onto grilled meat or fish.

1 bunch cilantro
6 tablespoons unsweetened shredded coconut
6 tablespoons toasted peanuts
½ jalapeño, serrano, or Thai chile (optional)
Juice of ½ lemon
1 tablespoon Garlic Oil (page 202)
1 tablespoon olive oil
Salt to taste

1. In a food processor, roughly chop the cilantro. Add the coconut, peanuts, chile (if using), and lemon juice, and process to a paste.

2. With the processor running, add the Garlic Oil and olive oil, and process until the desired texture has been achieved. If the mixture is too thick, add more oil or lemon juice or a bit of water. Taste and add salt as needed.

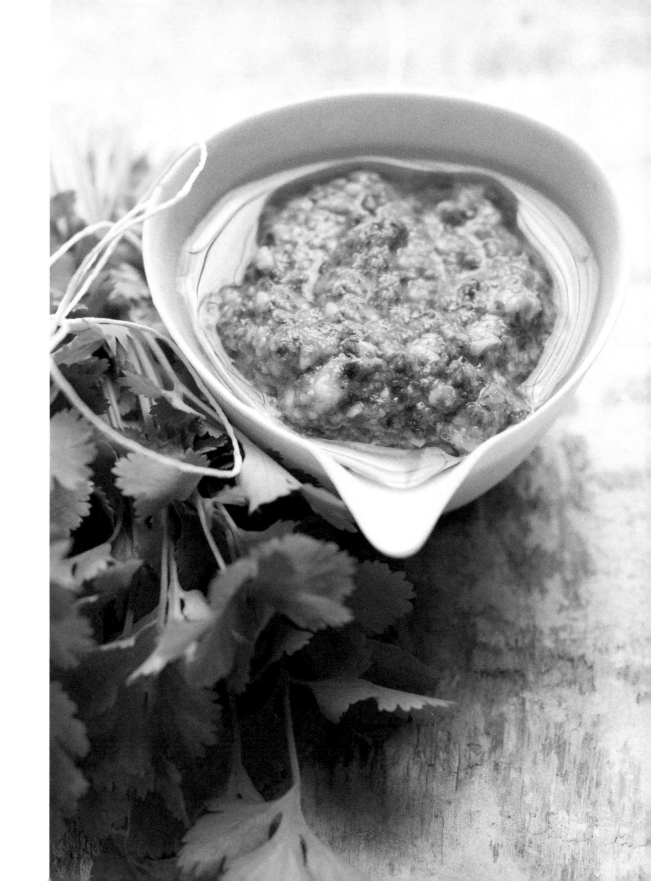

Pico de Gallo Salsa

MAKES ABOUT 2 CUPS

PREP TIME: 5 MINUTES, PLUS
15 MINUTES TO REST

COOK TIME: NONE

Cooking Tip: For a saucier consistency, place all of the ingredients in a food processor and pulse to a chunky or smooth purée as desired.

PER SERVING

(½ CUP)

Calories: 95
Protein: 2g
Total Fat: 7g
Saturated Fat: 1g
Carbohydrates: 8g
Fiber: 2g
Sodium: 300mg

This quick, simple salsa is the perfect accompaniment to a wide array of dishes, from Spiced Tortilla Chips (page 88), to Chipotle Tofu and Sweet Potato Tacos with Avocado Salsa (page 146), to Grilled Carne Asada Tacos with Chimichurri Sauce (page 172). Or use it to top any grilled meat or scrambled, fried, or poached eggs.

5 medium tomatoes, chopped
1 jalapeño chile, minced
½ cup minced fresh cilantro
Juice of 1 lime
2 tablespoons Garlic Oil (page 202)
2 tablespoons olive oil
½ teaspoon salt

1. In a medium bowl, combine all of the ingredients and toss to combine well.

2. Let sit at room temperature for 15 minutes. Serve immediately or store, covered, in the refrigerator for up to 3 days.

Thai Red Curry Paste

MAKES ABOUT ½ CUP

PREP TIME: 5 MINUTES,
PLUS 15 MINUTES TO
SOAK CHILES

COOK TIME: 1 MINUTE

Substitution Tip: For a
shellfish-free version,
substitute 2 teaspoons
fish sauce for the
shrimp paste.

PER SERVING

(1 TABLESPOON)

Calories: 23
Protein: 1g
Total Fat: 0g
Saturated Fat: 0g
Carbohydrates: 5g
Fiber: 1g
Sodium: 193mg

Store-bought Thai curry pastes are great for adding quick flavor to stir-fries or soups, but most contain high-FODMAP ingredients like garlic and shallots. This version omits those ingredients but doesn't skimp on flavor.

6 dry red chiles
1 teaspoon ground cumin
1 teaspoon ground coriander
1 teaspoon paprika
3-inch piece fresh ginger
2 (6-inch) pieces fresh lemongrass
2 tablespoons chopped fresh cilantro
2 teaspoons shrimp paste
2 Kaffir lime leaves
¼ teaspoon salt

1. Place the chiles in a heatproof bowl and cover them with boiling water. Let soak for 15 minutes, then drain.

2. Heat a medium skillet over medium-high heat, add the cumin, coriander, and paprika, and cook, stirring, for about 1 minute, until fragrant. Transfer the spices to a food processor.

3. Add the ginger, lemongrass, cilantro, shrimp paste, lime leaves, and salt to the food processor, along with the drained chiles. Process to a smooth paste.

4. Refrigerate in a sealed container for up to a week, or freeze for up to 3 months.

Thai Sweet Chili Sauce

MAKES ABOUT 1 CUP

PREP TIME: 5 MINUTES

COOK TIME: 7 MINUTES

Cooking Tip: The seeds are where much of a chile's heat is located, so leave the seeds in for a hotter version of this sauce. If you prefer a milder sauce, take them out before chopping the chiles.

PER SERVING

(2 TABLESPOONS)

Calories: 85
Protein: 0g
Total Fat: 0g
Saturated Fat: 0g
Carbohydrates: 20g
Fiber: 0g
Sodium: 582mg

An especially versatile condiment, Thai Sweet Chili Sauce makes a tasty dip for spring or summer rolls, cooked shrimp, or other seafood, as well as an excellent marinade or sauce for chicken or fish. Store-bought versions usually contain garlic, but this one doesn't, so to get that traditional flavor, just combine it with a bit of Garlic Oil (page 202).

1 cup plus 2 tablespoons water, divided
2 tablespoons cornstarch
2 tablespoons finely chopped chiles
  (use red jalapeños, red Thai, Fresno, or other red chiles)
⅔ cup sugar
⅓ cup rice vinegar
2 teaspoons salt

1. In a small bowl, stir together 2 tablespoons of the water and the cornstarch until smooth.

2. In a medium saucepan over medium heat, combine the remaining 1 cup water, chiles, sugar, vinegar, and salt, and bring to a boil. Reduce the heat to low and simmer, uncovered, until the sauce starts to become syrupy, about 5 minutes.

3. Give the cornstarch mixture a stir and whisk it into the simmering sauce. Cook, stirring, for 1 minute more, until the sauce is thickened. Remove from the heat and let cool slightly before using.

4. Store in a covered container in the refrigerator for up to a week.

Basil "Hollandaise" Sauce

MAKES ABOUT 1 ½ CUPS

PREP TIME: 5 MINUTES

COOK TIME: NONE

Cooking Tip: You want to use a lightly flavored oil for this recipe, so choose a light olive oil (not extra-virgin) or a neutral-flavored oil like grapeseed.

PER SERVING

(¼ CUP)

Calories: 161
Protein: 1g
Total Fat: 17g
Saturated Fat: 2g
Carbohydrates: 3g
Fiber: 0g
Sodium: 203mg

Classic Hollandaise sauce is rich with butter and egg yolks. This dairy-free and egg-free version is lighter but equally delicious. Serve it drizzled over roasted or steamed vegetables, poached eggs, chicken, or fish.

½ cup cold rice milk

½ cup fresh basil leaves

4 teaspoons lemon juice

1 tablespoon nutritional yeast

½ teaspoon salt

⅛ teaspoon cayenne pepper

⅛ teaspoon turmeric

¼ teaspoon xanthan gum

½ cup light olive oil

In a blender, combine the rice milk, basil, lemon juice, nutritional yeast, salt, cayenne, and turmeric, and process until smooth. Add the xanthan gum and blend on high until the mixture becomes foamy. With the blender running, slowly add the oil, blending until the sauce is thick.

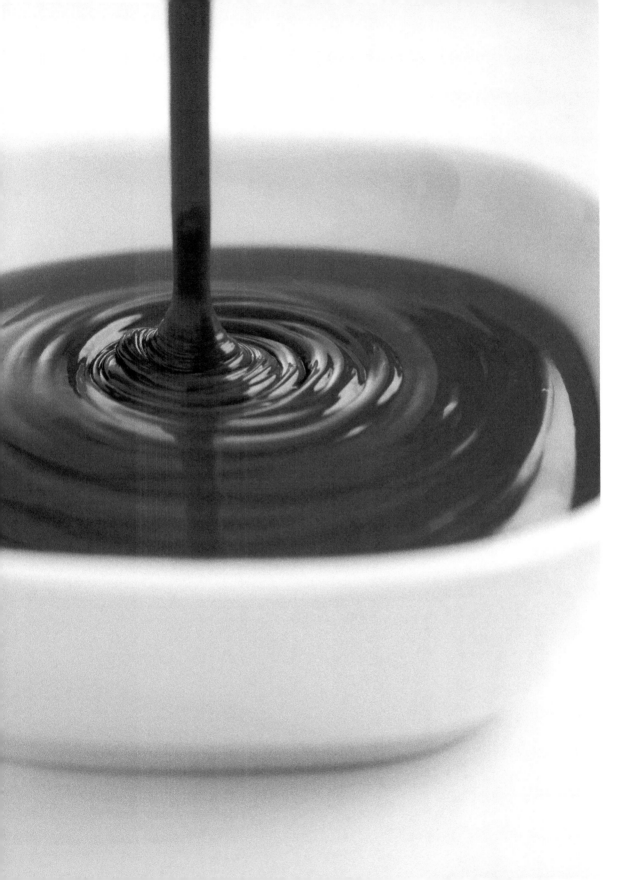

Luscious Hot Fudge Sauce

Substitution Tip: If you prefer, you can substitute coconut sugar or maple syrup for the granulated sugar, and use palm sugar instead of the brown sugar.

PER SERVING

(2 TABLESPOONS)

Calories: 135
Protein: 2g
Total Fat: 8g
Saturated Fat: 6g
Carbohydrates: 17g
Fiber: 1g
Sodium: 48mg

Made with coconut milk and dark chocolate, this rich, chocolaty sauce is divine drizzled over (dairy-free) ice cream or used as a dip for fruit. Make a jar of it to keep in the fridge for those times when you need a chocolate fix.

⅔ cup full-fat coconut milk
½ cup granulated sugar
⅓ cup brown sugar
¼ cup unsweetened cocoa powder
¼ teaspoon salt
6 ounces bittersweet chocolate (dairy-free and gluten-free), chopped, divided
2 tablespoons coconut oil
1 teaspoon vanilla extract

1. In a medium saucepan combine the coconut milk, sugars, cocoa powder, salt, and half of the chocolate, and bring to a boil. Reduce the heat to low and simmer, stirring occasionally, for 5 minutes.

2. Remove the pan from the heat and whisk in the remaining chocolate along with the coconut oil and vanilla. Stir until smooth.

3. Let cool for 15 to 20 minutes before serving. Serve warm or store in a covered container in the refrigerator for up to 2 weeks.

Tangy Lemon Curd

MAKES ABOUT 2 CUPS

PREP TIME: 5 MINUTES,
PLUS 4 HOURS TO CHILL

COOK TIME: 10 MINUTES

Substitution Tip: For a dairy-free version, replace the butter with a vegan butter substitute or coconut oil. For an egg-free version, omit the eggs and use a mixture of ¼ cup cornstarch dissolved in ¼ cup water, along with the butter, butter substitute, or coconut oil. Cook until the mixture thickens, for 3 to 4 minutes.

PER SERVING

(¼ CUP)

Calories: 240
Protein: 3g
Total Fat: 12.4g
Saturated Fat: 7.2g
Carbohydrates: 32g
Fiber: 2g
Sodium: 42mg

Rich and tangy lemon curd makes a delightful spread for (gluten-free) toast or scones, and it can also add intense lemony flavor to desserts like Gluten-Free Lemon-Filled Cookies (page 227).

1 cup granulated sugar
1 tablespoon finely grated lemon zest
1 cup lemon juice (from about 5 large lemons)
3 tablespoons chilled butter
3 eggs, lightly beaten

1. In a medium saucepan over medium heat, whisk together the sugar, lemon zest, and lemon juice. Whisk in the butter and eggs, and cook the mixture, stirring constantly (be careful not to let it come to a boil), until it becomes thick, for 8 to 10 minutes.

2. Transfer the mixture to a ramekin or custard bowl, and cover with plastic wrap, pressing the plastic directly onto the surface of the curd to prevent a skin from forming, and chill for 4 hours.

Whipped Coconut Cream

MAKES ABOUT 2 CUPS

PREP TIME: 10 MINUTES,
PLUS OVERNIGHT TO CHILL

COOK TIME: NONE

Ingredient Tip: If you can
find coconut cream, skip
the overnight refrigera-
tion and simply use 1 cup
of coconut cream instead.

PER SERVING

(¼ CUP)

Calories: 83
Protein: 1g
Total Fat: 7g
Saturated Fat: 6g
Carbohydrates: 5g
Fiber: 1g
Sodium: 5mg

Whipped cream is a divine topping for many desserts, from (dairy-free) ice cream sundaes to Strawberry-Rhubarb Crisp (page 238). This dairy-free version, made with coconut milk, is just as versatile.

1 can full-fat coconut milk, refrigerated overnight
2 tablespoons maple syrup
½ teaspoon vanilla extract

1. Carefully turn over the can of coconut milk and open the bottom of the can. Pour off the liquid coconut milk, leaving the thick cream (you should end up with about 1 cup of cream). Add some of the coconut milk, if needed, so that it equals 1 cup, saving the rest of the coconut milk for another purpose). Place the coconut cream in a large bowl and, using an electric mixer set on high speed, whip the cream until it becomes very fluffy and forms soft peaks.

2. Add the maple syrup and vanilla, and gently whip until just incorporated.

3. Refrigerate until ready to serve, or up to 3 days.

Easy Lemon Vinaigrette

MAKES ABOUT ⅔ CUP

PREP TIME: 5 MINUTES

COOK TIME: NONE

Cooking Tip: If you like a touch of garlicky flavor in your vinaigrette, substitute 2 tablespoons of Garlic Oil (page 202) for 2 tablespoons of the olive oil.

PER SERVING

(2 TABLESPOONS)

Calories: 125
Protein: 0g
Total Fat: 14g
Saturated Fat: 2g
Carbohydrates: 1g
Fiber: 0g
Sodium: 299mg

This simple lemon dressing is light and flavorful, perfect for tossing with a crisp green salad. It offers a nice balance that makes it ideal for bitter lettuces like endive or radicchio, too. Add shaved Parmesan cheese, if you like, for a salty finish.

1 teaspoon finely grated lemon zest
3 tablespoons lemon juice
1 teaspoon sugar
¾ teaspoon Dijon mustard
¾ teaspoon salt
¼ teaspoon freshly ground black pepper
6 tablespoons olive oil

1. Whisk the lemon zest, lemon juice, sugar, mustard, salt, and pepper together in a small bowl. While whisking, add the oil in a thin stream, whisking until the mixture thickens.

2. Use immediately or store in a covered container in the refrigerator for up to a week.

Maple-Mustard Vinaigrette

MAKES ABOUT ⅔ CUP

PREP TIME: 5 MINUTES

COOK TIME: NONE

Cooking Tip: For an especially festive fall salad, add toasted nuts, such as pecans or walnuts, or dried cranberries.

PER SERVING

(2 TABLESPOONS)

Calories: 142
Protein: 0g
Total Fat: 14g
Saturated Fat: 2g
Carbohydrates: 5g
Fiber: 0g
Sodium: 157mg

In this flavorful homemade dressing—a cinch to prepare—spicy Dijon mustard, sweet maple syrup, and tart balsamic vinegar mingle to create a perfectly balanced vinaigrette for any type of greens.

2 tablespoons balsamic vinegar
2 tablespoons maple syrup
2 tablespoons Dijon mustard
¼ teaspoon salt
¼ teaspoon freshly ground black pepper
6 tablespoons olive oil

1. Whisk the vinegar, maple syrup, mustard, salt, and pepper together in a small bowl. While whisking, add the oil in a thin stream, whisking until the mixture thickens.

2. Use immediately or store in a covered container in the refrigerator for up to a week.

Egg-Free Caesar Dressing

MAKES ABOUT ¾ CUP

PREP TIME: 5 MINUTES

COOK TIME: NONE

Cooking Tip: Canned anchovy fillets can be extremely salty. To eliminate some of the excess salt, rinse them in cold running water and pat dry with paper towels before using.

PER SERVING

(2 TABLESPOONS)

Calories: 229
Protein: 18g
Total Fat: 17g
Saturated Fat: 4g
Carbohydrates: 2g
Fiber: 0g
Sodium: 3632mg

This tangy, salty dressing; a pile of crisp romaine lettuce leaves; and a handful of gluten-free croutons are all you need to make a perfect salad to start off a special meal. Or add a bit of grilled chicken breast to turn this salad into a meal in and of itself. You can leave out the anchovies, if you like; just add a bit more salt to compensate.

4 whole anchovy fillets
2 tablespoons Dijon mustard
1 tablespoon red-wine vinegar
1 teaspoon gluten-free soy sauce or coconut aminos
Juice of ½ lemon
¼ teaspoon salt
¼ teaspoon freshly ground black pepper
¼ cup olive oil
¼ cup Garlic Oil (page 202)
¼ cup freshly grated Parmesan cheese

1. In a blender or food processor, combine the anchovies, mustard, vinegar, soy sauce or coconut aminos, lemon juice, salt, and pepper. Pulse to chop the anchovies and combine well.

2. With the processor running, slowly add the olive oil and Garlic Oil in a thin stream. Process until the mixture is thickened. Add the cheese and pulse just to incorporate.

3. Serve immediately or store in a covered container in the refrigerator for up to a week.

Low-FODMAP Spicy Ketchup

MAKES ABOUT 1½ CUPS

PREP TIME: 5 MINUTES

COOK TIME: 20 MINUTES

Cooking Tip: For a milder version, omit or reduce the cayenne. For an alternative flavor, replace the spices with 1 to 2 teaspoons curry powder or chili powder.

PER SERVING

(2 TABLESPOONS)

Calories: 28
Protein: 1g
Total Fat: 0g
Saturated Fat: 0g
Carbohydrates: 7g
Fiber: 1g
Sodium: 289mg

Whereas store-bought ketchup is flavored with garlic and onions, this version uses Garlic Oil (page 202) to add a base of garlicky flavor without the FODMAPs. This spicy ketchup will dress up everything from French fries to Crunchy Homemade Fish Sticks (page 180).

2 tablespoons Garlic Oil (page 202)
¼ cup tomato paste
¼ cup light-brown sugar
½ teaspoon ground ginger
¼ teaspoon cayenne
¼ teaspoon ground allspice
⅛ teaspoon ground cinnamon
⅛ teaspoon ground cloves
¼ cup red-wine vinegar
1 (15-ounce) can tomato sauce
½ teaspoon salt
¼ teaspoon freshly ground black pepper

1. Heat the Garlic Oil in a small saucepan over medium heat. Add the tomato paste and cook, stirring, for 1 minute.

2. Add the sugar, ginger, cayenne, allspice, cinnamon, and cloves, and cook, stirring frequently, until the sugar is fully dissolved. Stir in the vinegar, tomato sauce, salt, and pepper. Cook, stirring occasionally, for 15 to 20 minutes, until the sauce is very thick.

3. Let cool to room temperature. Serve immediately or store in a covered container in the refrigerator for up to a week.

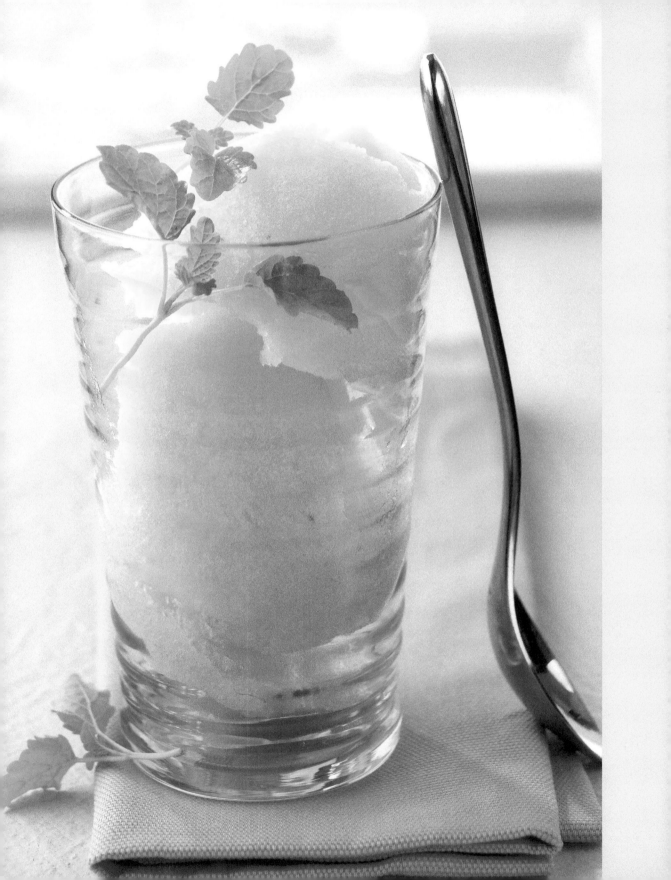

11

Desserts and Sweets

Raspberry-Chia Seed Ice Pops

MAKES 6 ICE POPS

PREP TIME: 10 MINUTES,
PLUS 5 HOURS TO FREEZE

COOK TIME: NONE

Cooking Tip: If you feel lazy or don't want to wait so long for your pops, combine all of the ingredients in the blender, pour into the molds, and freeze for 4 hours.

PER SERVING

Calories: 115
Protein: 1g
Total Fat: 6g
Saturated Fat: 0g
Carbohydrates: 14g
Fiber: 3g
Sodium: 16mg

These refreshing ice pops are lightly sweetened with sugar and are rich with coconut milk. Make up a batch the next time the mercury rises, and you'll be glad you did. Feel free to mix or substitute other berries, such as blueberries or strawberries, for variety.

1½ cup raspberries (fresh or thawed frozen)
4 tablespoons sugar, divided
½ cup water
6 ice-pop molds and handles
1 (15-ounce) can light coconut milk
1½ tablespoons chia seeds

1. In a blender, combine the raspberries, 2 tablespoons of the sugar, and water and blend until smooth.

2. Fill each ice-pop mold with about 1 inch of the raspberry mixture, and place in the freezer to harden (about 30 minutes). Place the remaining raspberry mixture in the refrigerator.

3. Whisk together the coconut milk, the remaining 2 tablespoons sugar, and the chia seeds in a small bowl.

4. Add the coconut milk mixture to the ice-pop molds, distributing evenly. Freeze for another 30 minutes.

5. Add the remaining raspberry mixture to the ice-pop molds, add the sticks or handles, and freeze for at least 4 hours, until completely frozen solid.

Pineapple Sorbet

SERVES 6

PREP TIME: 10 MINUTES,
PLUS SEVERAL HOURS TO
FREEZE AND CHILL

COOK TIME: NONE

Cooking Tip: If you don't
have an ice cream maker,
no problem: Just freeze
the sorbet in a baking
dish for 2 to 3 hours, stir
it up, and continue to
freeze, stirring every
30 minutes or so to break
up any ice chunks, for
another 3 to 4 hours.

PER SERVING

Calories: 181
Protein: 1g
Total Fat: 0g
Saturated Fat: 0g
Carbohydrates: 48g
Fiber: 2g
Sodium: 2mg

Three ingredients are all you need to make this refreshing tropical treat. If you don't have fresh pineapple, substitute 4 cups diced unsweetened canned pineapple.

1 small pineapple, peeled, cored, and cut into chunks
2 tablespoons lemon juice
1 cup sugar

1. In a food processor, combine the pineapple and lemon juice, and process to a smooth purée. Add the sugar and process for another 1 to 2 minutes, until the sugar is completely dissolved.

2. Transfer the mixture to an ice cream maker and freeze according to the manufacturer's instructions.

3. Transfer to a freezer-safe container and freeze for several hours until very firm. Serve frozen.

Dairy-Free Coffee Ice Cream

SERVES 6

PREP TIME: 5 MINUTES,
PLUS SEVERAL HOURS TO
CHILL AND SEVERAL HOURS
TO FREEZE

COOK TIME: 5 MINUTES

Cooking Tip: If you don't have an ice cream maker, no problem: Just freeze the ice cream in a baking dish for 2 to 3 hours, stir it up, and continue to freeze, stirring every 30 minutes or so to break up any ice chunks, for another 3 to 4 hours.

PER SERVING

Calories: 357
Protein: 2g
Total Fat: 26g
Saturated Fat: 21g
Carbohydrates: 30g
Fiber: 0g
Sodium: 36mg

Just four ingredients make this simple ice cream perfectly dreamy. Try it in a sundae topped with Luscious Hot Fudge Sauce (page 213) and Whipped Coconut Cream (page 215).

2 (15-ounce) cans full-fat coconut milk
¾ cup granulated sugar
¾ strong brewed coffee
1½ teaspoons vanilla extract

1. In a medium saucepan set over medium heat, whisk together the coconut milk, sugar, and coffee, and heat for about 5 minutes, until the sugar is dissolved. Remove from the heat and stir in the vanilla.

2. Transfer to a bowl and chill, covered, in the refrigerator for several hours or overnight.

3. Transfer the mixture to an ice cream maker and freeze according to the manufacturer's instructions.

4. Transfer to a freezer-safe container and freeze for several hours until very firm. Serve frozen.

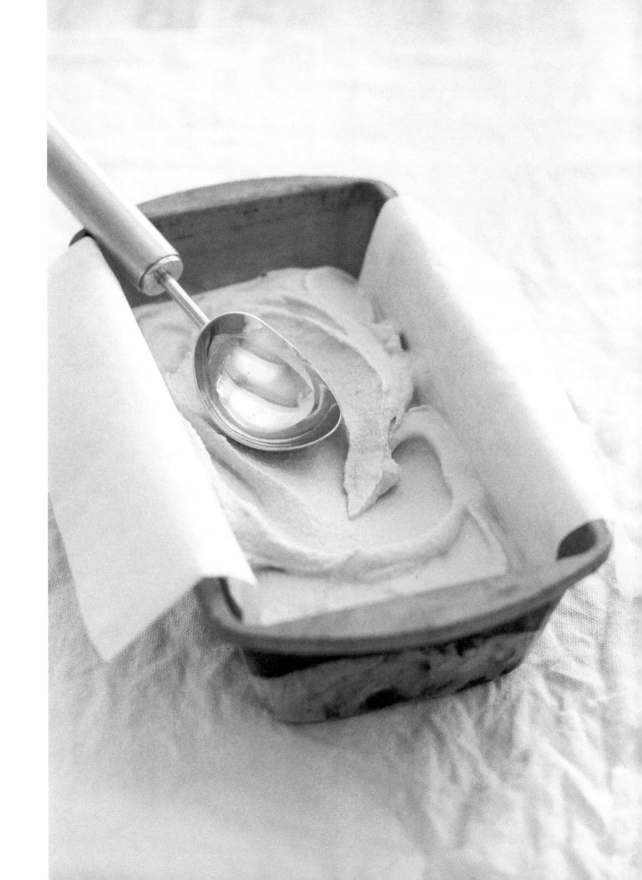

No-Bake Coconut Cookie Bars

MAKES ABOUT 12 BARS

PREP TIME: 5 MINUTES,
PLUS 1 HOUR TO CHILL

COOK TIME: NONE

Cooking Tip: To speed
up the chilling process,
freeze the bars for
15 minutes.

PER SERVING

Calories: 122
Protein: 1g
Total Fat: 9g
Saturated Fat: 8g
Carbohydrates: 11g
Fiber: 1g
Sodium: 54mg

Containing just a handful of ingredients, these addictive coconut bars couldn't be simpler to prepare. They're lightly sweetened with maple syrup, which also adds great flavor, and you can have a batch ready in no time. Kids and adults alike will love snacking on them.

2 cups shredded unsweetened coconut
½ cup maple syrup
¼ cup coconut oil
1 teaspoon vanilla extract
¼ teaspoon salt

1. Combine all of the ingredients in a food processor and process to combine well.

2. Transfer the mixture to a baking dish or rectangular cake pan (8-by-11-inch or similar capacity), and chill in the refrigerator for 1 hour.

3. Cut into 12 bars and serve chilled.

Gluten-Free Lemon-Filled Cookies

MAKES ABOUT 20 COOKIES

PREP TIME: 15 MINUTES

COOK TIME: 12 MINUTES

PER SERVING

Calories: 306
Protein: 2g
Total Fat: 21g
Saturated Fat: 17g
Carbohydrates: 26g
Fiber: 4g
Sodium: 56mg

These flavorful cookies are easy to prepare, especially if you already have the Tangy Lemon Curd (page 214) on hand. These cookies are a treat for the taste buds as well as the eyes, a delightfully simple sugar cookie with a glistening, lemony filling peeking out from the cut-out center.

1 cup sugar
1 cup unsalted butter, softened
2 egg yolks
1½ teaspoons vanilla extract
2¼ cups gluten-free flour (low-FODMAP blend)
¼ teaspoon salt
1 cup Tangy Lemon Curd (page 214)

1. In a large bowl, cream together the sugar and butter using an electric mixer set at medium speed, about 3 minutes. Add the egg yolks and vanilla and continue beating on medium speed for about 2 minutes more. Add the flour and salt and beat with the mixer set on low until the dry ingredients are incorporated, about 1 minute. Cover the bowl and chill the dough in the refrigerator for 1 hour.

2. When the dough is well chilled and firm, remove it from the refrigerator and preheat the oven to 350°F.

3. Split the dough into two pieces and, working with one piece at a time, turn it out onto a lightly floured (using a suitable gluten-free flour, of course) work surface. Roll the dough out to a thickness of about ¼ inch. Cut the dough into circles using a round cookie cutter. Using a smaller cookie cutter—this could be a smaller circle or a star, heart, or other shape—cut out the center of half of the circles. Ball up the leftover dough, including the small cutout pieces, and repeat the process until all of the dough is used. ▶

4. Arrange the cookies on a baking sheet and bake in the preheated oven for about 8 to 12 minutes, until they are very lightly browned and crisp. Transfer the cookies to a cooling rack and cool completely.

5. Spread the lemon curd on the whole-circle cookies and top with the cutout cookies. Serve at room temperature.

Chocolate-Walnut Haystacks

MAKES ABOUT 12 COOKIES

PREP TIME: 10 MINUTES,
PLUS 30 MINUTES TO CHILL

COOK TIME: 2 MINUTES

Substitution Tip: For a nut-free version, substitute ¾ cup puffed rice cereal for the walnuts.

PER SERVING

Calories: 113
Protein: 3g
Total Fat: 10g
Saturated Fat: 5g
Carbohydrates: 5g
Fiber: 1g
Sodium: 6mg

These chocolaty and nutty no-bake treats make a great afternoon snack or after-dinner sweet. This version calls for walnuts, but you can substitute any nuts you like; try pecans, almonds, hazelnuts, or even macadamia nuts for a tropical flavor that pairs well with the coconut.

2 ounces dark chocolate (gluten-free, dairy-free)
1 tablespoon coconut oil
½ cup unsweetened coconut flakes
¾ cup chopped walnut pieces

1. Line a baking sheet with parchment paper.

2. In the top of a double boiler set over simmering water, or in a microwave, melt the chocolate and coconut oil together.

3. In a medium bowl, combine the coconut flakes and walnuts. Stir in the melted chocolate mixture until well combined.

4. Drop the mixture onto the prepared baking sheet by rounded spoonfuls. Refrigerate until set, at least 30 minutes. Serve chilled.

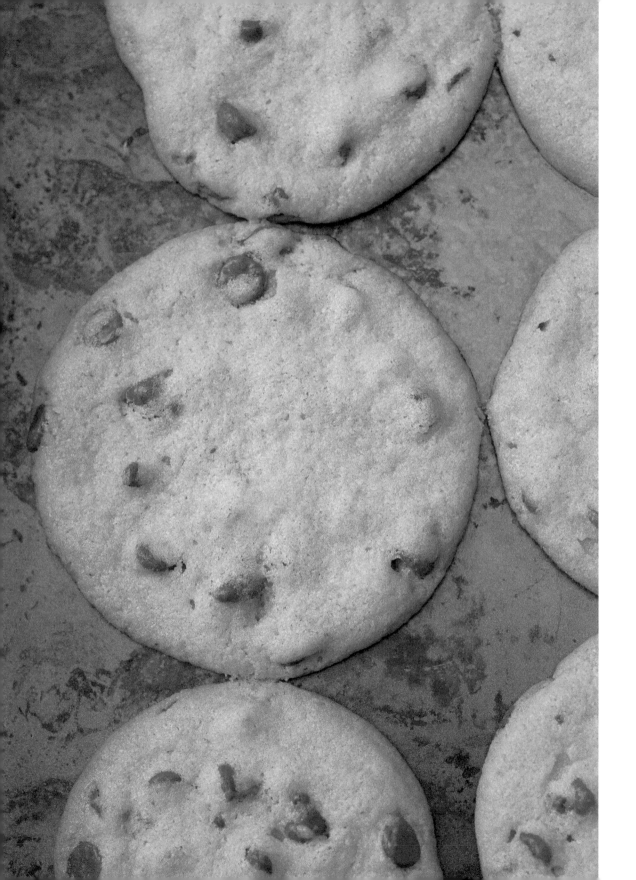

Crispy Gluten-Free Chocolate Chip Cookies

MAKES ABOUT 24 COOKIES

PREP TIME: 10 MINUTES

COOK TIME: 10 MINUTES

Substitution Tip: For an egg-free version, substitute a chia-seed egg replacer: Grind 1 tablespoon white chia-seed meal in a food processor or spice grinder, and mix with 3 tablespoons warm water. Let the mixture stand for 5 to 10 minutes, until it thickens to the consistency of raw eggs. To make these cookies dairy-free, replace the butter with coconut oil or vegan margarine.

PER SERVING

Calories: 126
Protein: 1g
Total Fat: 7g
Saturated Fat: 4g
Carbohydrates: 16g
Fiber: 1g
Sodium: 112mg

These simple cookies are the perfect treat, a gluten-free and low-FODMAP version of everyone's childhood favorite. For a festive mint-chocolate holiday version, add a teaspoon of peppermint extract along with the vanilla extract.

1 cup plus 2 tablespoons gluten-free flour (low-FODMAP blend such as King Arthur's)
½ teaspoon gluten-free baking powder
½ teaspoon gluten-free baking soda
½ teaspoon salt
½ cup butter, at room temperature
¼ cup sugar
½ cup packed light brown sugar
1 teaspoon vanilla extract
1 egg
1 cup semisweet chocolate chips

1. Preheat the oven to 350°F.

2. Line a large baking sheet with parchment paper.

3. In a medium bowl, combine the flour, baking powder, baking soda, and salt.

4. In a large bowl using an electric mixer or in the bowl of a stand mixer, cream the butter and sugars together, mixing on medium speed, until well combined. ▶

5. Add the egg and vanilla and beat to incorporate. Add the flour mixture in 2 additions, beating to incorporate after each addition. Stir in the chocolate chips.

6. Drop the cookies onto the prepared baking sheet by rounded spoonfuls, leaving at least 2 inches of space between them (you will need to bake in two batches or use two baking sheets).

7. Bake in the preheated oven for 10 minutes. Let the cookies cool on the baking sheet for 3 or 4 minutes before transferring them to a wire rack to cool completely.

Crunchy Peanut Butter Cookies

MAKES ABOUT 18 COOKIES

PREP TIME: 10 MINUTES

COOK TIME: 10 MINUTES

Substitution Tip: For an egg-free version, substitute a chia-seed egg replacer: Grind 1 tablespoon white chia-seed meal in a food processor or spice grinder, and mix with 3 tablespoons warm water. Let the mixture stand for 5 to 10 minutes, until it thickens to the consistency of raw eggs. To make these cookies nut-free, replace the peanut butter with sunflower-seed butter.

PER SERVING

Calories: 135
Protein: 4g
Total Fat: 7g
Saturated Fat: 1g
Carbohydrates: 14g
Fiber: 1g
Sodium: 16mg

With only five ingredients, this is one of the simplest cookie recipes ever. Rest assured, though, that these will quickly become a favorite for anyone who tastes them. These crunchy, nutty cookies, with just the right level of sweetness, are perfectly addictive.

1 cup all-natural peanut butter
1 cup sugar
1 teaspoon vanilla extract
1 egg, lightly beaten
Pinch salt

1. Preheat the oven to 350°F.

2. In a medium bowl, combine the peanut butter, sugar, vanilla, egg, and salt, and mix well. Drop the mixture by rounded spoonfuls onto an ungreased baking sheet, leaving about 1 inch of space between the cookies. Using the back of a fork, flatten the cookies, making a crosshatch pattern with the fork tines.

3. Bake in the preheated oven for about 10 minutes, until the edges of the cookies begin to turn golden brown. Transfer the cookies to a wire rack to cool. Serve at room temperature.

Triple-Berry Shortcakes

MAKES 6 CAKES

PREP TIME: 15 MINUTES

COOK TIME: 15 MINUTES

Substitution Tip: For a dairy-free version, substitute coconut oil for the butter and Whipped Coconut Cream (see recipe page 215) for the whipped heavy cream.

PER SERVING

Calories: 318
Protein: 3g
Total Fat: 17g
Saturated Fat: 10g
Carbohydrates: 41g
Fiber: 3g
Sodium: 86mg

This classic dessert is best prepared in the early summer, at the height of berry season. Using all three berries creates the perfect Fourth of July dessert, but you can opt to use just one type of berry or substitute other fruits as availability varies.

¼ cup butter
½ cup plus 2 tablespoons powdered sugar, divided
2 eggs
½ teaspoon vanilla extract
½ cup cornstarch
¾ teaspoon baking powder
1 cup sliced strawberries
1 cup blueberries
1 cup raspberries
1 cup heavy cream
¼ cup maple syrup

1. Preheat the oven to 375°F and spray 6 muffin cups with cooking spray.

2. In a large bowl cream butter and ½ cup sugar together using an electric mixer set on medium speed. Add the eggs and vanilla and beat until the mixture is pale yellow and fluffy.

3. In a small bowl, combine the cornstarch and baking powder, and add it a little at a time to the butter mixture. Beat until well combined.

4. Scoop the mixture into the prepared muffin cups, filing each about halfway.

5. Bake in the preheated oven for about 15 minutes, or until a toothpick inserted into the center comes out clean.

6. Remove from the pan from the oven and transfer the cakes to a rack to cool.

7. In a medium bowl, combine the berries and toss together gently.

8. In another medium bowl, whip the cream with an electric mixer until fluffy and soft peaks form. Add the remaining 2 tablespoons of sugar and beat until incorporated.

9. Split the cakes and place them in wide shallow bowls. Top with the berries and whipped cream to serve.

Cinnamon-Coconut Rice Pudding

SERVES 4

PREP TIME: 5 MINUTES

COOK TIME: 40 MINUTES

Substitution Tip: For a
dairy-free version, replace
the lactose-free milk with
additional coconut milk
or rice milk.

PER SERVING

Calories: 261
Protein: 4g
Total Fat: 5g
Saturated Fat: 4g
Carbohydrates: 50g
Fiber: 1g
Sodium: 183mg

This simple, lightly sweetened, spiced pudding is comfort in a bowl. The coconut milk gives it a hint of tropical flavor, but the overall effect is of the same old-fashioned rice pudding you remember from childhood. Serve as is or dress it up with fresh or dried fruit as you see fit.

1½ cups cold cooked rice
1 cup lactose-free milk
2½ cups coconut milk
⅓ cup sugar
¼ teaspoon salt
¾ teaspoon ground cinnamon
½ teaspoon vanilla extract

1. In a medium saucepan, combine the rice, milk, coconut milk, sugar, and salt, and cook, uncovered, over medium heat, stirring frequently, for about 40 minutes, until the mixture thickens.

2. Remove from the heat, stir in the cinnamon and vanilla, and serve warm.

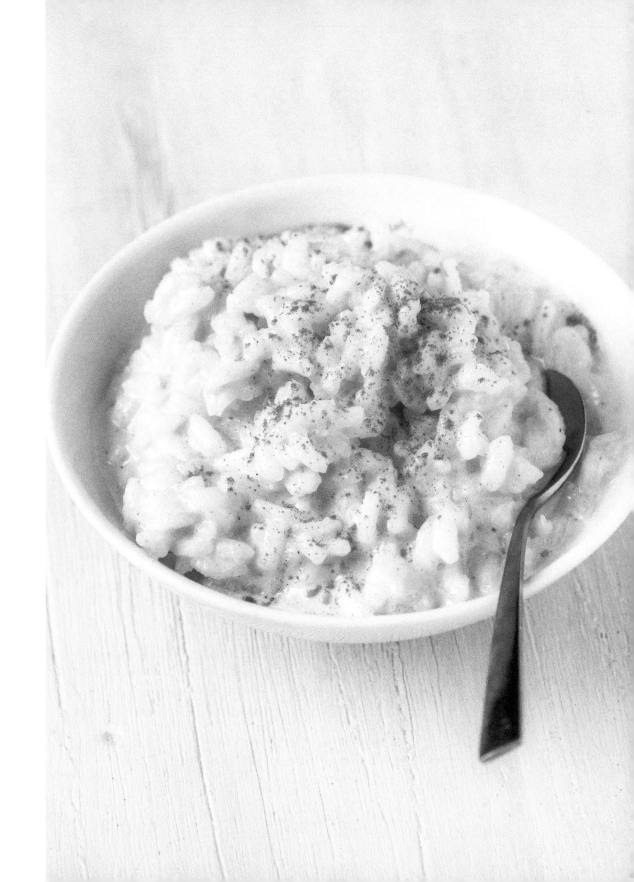

Strawberry-Rhubarb Crisp with Oat-Pecan Topping

SERVES 6

PREP TIME: 10 MINUTES

COOK TIME: 40 MINUTES

Substitution Tip: For a dairy-free version, replace the butter with coconut oil. For a nut-free version, use shredded, unsweetened coconut instead of pecans.

PER SERVING

Calories: 277
Protein: 4g
Total Fat: 14g
Saturated Fat: 6g
Carbohydrates: 38g
Fiber: 4g
Sodium: 115mg

Fruit crisp is a go-to, easy dessert you can make throughout the year. This version combines sweet strawberries and tart rhubarb, but you can substitute blueberries or raspberries based on what is in season.

FOR THE FILLING
Butter or coconut oil for preparing the pan
2 cups sliced strawberries
1 cup finely chopped rhubarb
¼ cup sugar
⅛ teaspoon salt

FOR THE TOPPING
1 cup gluten-free rolled oats
½ cup gluten-free oat flour
½ cup roughly chopped pecans
¼ cup packed light-brown sugar
Pinch salt
4 tablespoons cold unsalted butter

1. Preheat the oven to 350°F.

2. Grease a baking dish or 9-inch pie dish with butter or coconut oil.

3. In a medium bowl, combine the strawberries, rhubarb, sugar, and salt, and stir to mix. Transfer the mixture to the prepared baking dish.

4. To make the topping, combine the oats, oat flour, pecans, brown sugar, and salt in a medium bowl. Add the butter and mix with your hands until the butter is incorporated. Transfer the topping to the dish with the fruit, spreading it in an even layer over the top.

5. Bake in the preheated oven until the top is lightly browned and the filling is bubbly, for 35 to 40 minutes.

Caramelized Upside-Down Banana Cake

SERVES 8

PREP TIME: 10 MINUTES

COOK TIME: 25 MINUTES

Substitution Tip: For a dairy-free version, replace the butter with coconut oil. For an egg-free version, use a chia-seed egg replacer: Grind 2 tablespoons white chia-seed meal in a food processor or spice grinder, and mix with 6 tablespoons warm water. Let the mixture stand for 5 to 10 minutes, until it thickens to the consistency of raw eggs.

PER SERVING

Calories: 173
Protein: 3g
Total Fat: 7g
Saturated Fat: 5g
Carbohydrates: 26g
Fiber: 3g
Sodium: 130mg

While this cake bakes, the hidden bottom layer (soon to become the luscious top layer) of bananas caramelizes in a bath of melted butter and brown sugar, infusing the cake with an irresistibly rich sweetness. Once you invert the cake, the caramel seeps down, making this already-moist cake even more so.

Butter or coconut oil for preparing the pan
2 tablespoons unsalted butter
2 tablespoons brown sugar
2 bananas, 1 sliced and 1 mashed, divided
2 eggs, lightly beaten
⅓ cup maple syrup
¼ cup unsweetened coconut milk
1 teaspoon vanilla extract
½ teaspoon baking soda
1 teaspoon distilled vinegar
⅓ cup coconut flour

1. Preheat the oven to 350°F.

2. Grease a 9-inch cake pan with butter or coconut oil. Put the butter in the cake pan and place the pan in the oven for a few minutes while it is preheating. Once the butter is melted, remove the pan from the oven and tilt it around so that the butter thoroughly coats the bottom of the pan. Sprinkle the brown sugar over the melted butter and arrange the banana slices in the pan on top of the butter and sugar.

3. In a large bowl, combine the eggs, maple syrup, coconut milk, vanilla, baking soda, vinegar, and mashed banana, and mix well. Add the coconut flour, and stir to mix and eliminate any clumps. ▶

4. Pour the batter on top of the banana slices in the pan and spread into an even layer.

5. Bake in the preheated oven until the top of the cake is lightly browned and the cake is set in the center, for about 25 minutes. Remove from the oven and cool completely in the pan on a wire rack.

6. Slide a butter knife around the edge of the cake to loosen it from the pan, then invert the cake onto a serving platter. Serve at room temperature.

Chocolate Peanut Butter Cups

MAKES 8 CUPS

PREP TIME: 10 MINUTES,
PLUS 30 MINUTES TO FREEZE

COOK TIME: NONE

Substitution Tip: For a nut-free version, replace the peanut butter with sunflower seed butter.

PER SERVING

Calories: 312
Protein: 10g
Total Fat: 23g
Saturated Fat: 8g
Carbohydrates: 19g
Fiber: 2g
Sodium: 140mg

Peanut butter and chocolate is always a winning combination. These homemade chocolate peanut butter cups are sweetened with maple syrup and made with gluten-free, dairy-free dark chocolate, so there's nothing to stop you from savoring these sweet little treats.

1 cup all-natural creamy peanut butter
2 tablespoons coconut oil
2 tablespoons maple syrup
Pinch salt
1 cup gluten-free, dairy-free, dark chocolate chips

1. In a food processor, combine the peanut butter, coconut oil, maple syrup, and salt, and process until smooth and well combined. Spoon the mixture into cups of a mini muffin tin, dividing equally.

2. In the top of a double boiler set over simmering water, or in a microwave, melt the chocolate chips. Pour the melted chocolate over the peanut butter mixture in the muffin cups. Freeze for at least 30 minutes.

3. Pop the cups out of the muffin tin, using the tip of a sharp knife. Keep frozen until serving time, letting the cups sit at room temperature for 5 minutes before serving.

Chocolate Lava Cakes

MAKES 4 INDIVIDUAL CAKES

PREP TIME: 10 MINUTES

COOK TIME: 15 MINUTES

Substitution Tip: For a dairy-free version, replace the butter with coconut oil or a vegan butter substitute. For an egg-free version, substitute ½ cup of coconut milk and a chia-seed egg replacer: Grind 2 tablespoons white chia-seed meal in a food processor or spice grinder, and mix with 6 tablespoons warm water. Let the mixture stand for 5 to 10 minutes, until it thickens to the consistency of raw eggs.

PER SERVING

Calories: 415
Protein: 7g
Total Fat: 27g
Saturated Fat: 16g
Carbohydrates: 38g
Fiber: 2g
Sodium: 146mg

It doesn't get any better than rich, delicious, individual-size chocolate cakes. Oh, unless you add an ooey-gooey, melty, chocolaty center. But come to think of it, the best thing about this decadent cake might just be what a snap it is to make.

4 tablespoons unsalted butter, plus more for preparing the ramekins
5 ounces dark chocolate, chopped
2 eggs
2 egg yolks
¼ cup granulated sugar
½ teaspoon vanilla extract
3 tablespoons gluten-free all-purpose flour
⅛ teaspoon xanthan gum
1 tablespoon unsweetened cocoa powder
⅛ teaspoon salt
Powdered sugar, whipped cream, or Whipped Coconut Cream (page 215) for serving (optional)

1. Preheat the oven to 425°F.

2. Butter the insides of 4 (4-ounce) oven-safe ramekins and place the ramekins in a baking dish.

3. In the top of a double boiler set over simmering water, combine the chocolate and 4 tablespoons butter, stirring frequently, until melted.

4. In a large bowl, whisk together the eggs, egg yolks, sugar, and vanilla until the mixture becomes thick and very pale yellow. While whisking, slowly add the melted chocolate-butter mixture to the egg mixture until well combined.

5. Stir in the flour, xanthan gum, cocoa powder, and salt. Transfer the mixture to the prepared ramekins in the baking dish, dividing equally.

6. Place the baking dish in the preheated oven and add water to the baking dish so that it comes halfway up the sides of the ramekins. Bake for about 15 minutes, until the centers of the cakes are just barely set.

7. Carefully remove the ramekins from the baking dish and transfer them to a wire rack. Cool for about 10 minutes. Before serving, run a butter knife around the edge of each cake to loosen it from the ramekin and then invert it onto a serving plate. Serve immediately, with a dusting of powdered sugar or a dollop of whipped cream or Whipped Coconut Cream.

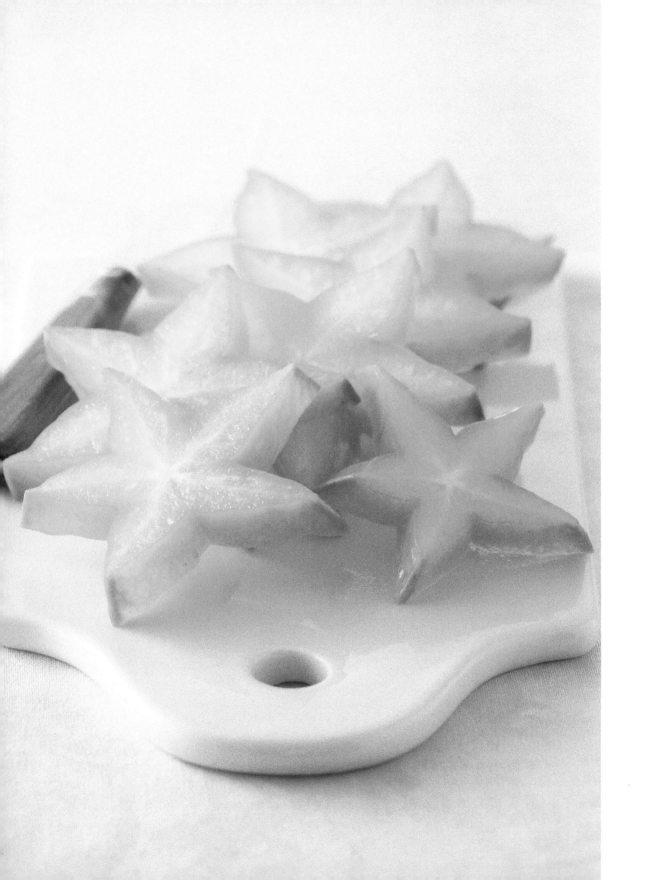

FODMAP Food Lists

COMMON SOURCES OF FODMAPS

FODMAP Type	Examples
Monosaccharides (Fructose)	agave nectar, apples, asparagus, cherries, fruit juice, high-fructose corn syrup (HFCS), honey, pears, sugar snap peas, watermelon
Disaccharides (Lactose)	cow's milk, goat's milk, heavy cream, ice cream, sheep's milk, soft cheeses (such as ricotta and cottage cheese), sour cream, yogurt
Oligosaccharides (Fructans)	artichokes, asparagus, barley, beets, Brussels sprouts, chicory, couscous, dandelion greens, garlic, graham flour, leeks, okra, onions, pasta, persimmons, rye, shallots, watermelon, wheat
Oligosaccharides (GOS)	chickpeas (garbanzo beans, not canned), hummus, kidney beans, lentils (not canned), peas, pinto beans, soybeans (whole)
Polyols	apples, apricots, avocados, blackberries, cauliflower, cherries, glycerol, isomalt, lactitol, lychees, maltitol, mannitol, mushrooms, nectarines, peaches, pears, plums, prunes, sorbitol, xylitol

FOODS TO ENJOY AND AVOID

The following table will help you make sense of which foods contain high doses of FODMAPs and which do not. Use this chart as a handy reference when planning shopping trips, meals, and snacks. Do keep in mind, however, that all produce contains some FODMAPs, so it's advisable to eat a wide variety of foods but limit most produce to one serving per meal (for example, ¾ cup cantaloupe or honeydew, 1 small banana, or 1 cup green beans). For everyday reference, the Monash University Low-FODMAP Diet app is an excellent source of information on the FODMAP content of different foods (www.med.monash.edu/cecs/gastro/fodmap/iphone-app.html).

Food Group	Foods to Eliminate (High-FODMAP)	Foods to Enjoy in Moderation (Moderate-FODMAP)	Foods to Enjoy (1 serving per meal) (Low-FODMAP)

FRUITS	apples
	apricots
	blackberries
	boysenberries
	cherries
	currants
	dates
	figs
	fruit juice
	grapefruit
	lychees
	mangos
	nectarines
	peaches
	pears
	persimmons
	plums
	prunes
	watermelon
		avocados
		  (⅛ medium avocado)
		banana chips
		  (10 chips)
		cranberries, dried
		  (1 tablespoon)
		grapefruit
		  (½ medium
		  grapefruit)
		pomegranate
		  (1 small pomegranate
		  or ¼ cup seeds)
		raisins
		  (1 tablespoon)
			bananas
			blueberries
			cantaloupe
			clementines
			cranberries
			fresh grapes
			honeydew
			kiwifruit
			lemons
			limes
			oranges
			papaya
			passionfruit
			pineapple
			raspberries
			rhubarb
			starfruit
			strawberries
			tangerines

FOODS TO ENJOY AND AVOID ▸

Food Group	Foods to Eliminate (High-FODMAP)	Foods to Enjoy in Moderation (Moderate-FODMAP)	Foods to Enjoy (1 serving per meal) (Low-FODMAP)
VEGETABLES	artichokes asparagus beets cauliflower chicory root fresh corn garlic scallions (white part) leeks (white part) mushrooms okra onions peas scallions (white part) shallots sugar snap peas	artichoke hearts 　(⅛ cup) broccoli (½ cup) Brussels sprouts 　(½ cup) butternut squash 　(¼ cup) canned corn (½ cup) celery (2½-inch stalk) green cabbage (1 cup) radicchio (1 cup) savoy cabbage (½ cup) sweet potatoes (½ cup) tomato 　(1 tomato per meal)	alfalfa sprouts bean sprouts bell peppers bok choy carrots chard chiles cucumbers eggplants endive fennel green beans kale leeks (green part) lettuce olives parsnips potatoes scallions (green part) spinach summer squash turnips
STARCHES AND LEGUMES	barley couscous hummus kidney beans lima beans pinto beans rye soybeans wheat wheat flour 　(including foods 　made with wheat 　flour—breads, 　pasta, cereal, etc.)	buckwheat kernels 　(⅛ cup) canned chickpeas 　(¼ cup) gluten-free oats 　(¼ cup dry or 　½ cup cooked) canned lentils (½ cup) sourdough spelt bread 　(2 slices)	arrowroot cornmeal gluten-free cornbread 　and corn tortillas gluten-free breads gluten-free flour gluten-free pasta millet polenta quinoa rice sorghum spelt tapioca tofu tempeh

▶ FOODS TO ENJOY AND AVOID

Food Group	Foods to Eliminate (High-FODMAP)	Foods to Enjoy in Moderation (Moderate-FODMAP)	Foods to Enjoy (1 serving per meal) (Low-FODMAP)

DAIRY	buttermilk
	cottage cheese
	custard
	ice cream
	milk
	  (cow, goat, sheep)
	pudding
	soft cheeses
	  (such as ricotta and
	  cream cheese)
	sour cream
	soy milk
	yogurt
		Brie
		feta cheese
		mozzarella cheese
		hard cheeses
		  (such as Parmesan,
		  cheddar, and Swiss;
		  1 ounce)
		half-and-half (¼ cup)
		heavy cream (½ cup)
			butter
			coconut milk
			lactose-free cow's milk
			rice milk
			whipped cream

NUTS AND SEEDS	cashews pistachios	almonds (10 nuts) flaxseed (1 tablespoon) hazelnuts (10 nuts)	Brazil nuts chia seeds macadamia nuts peanuts peanut butter pecans pine nuts sesame seeds sunflower seeds walnuts

MEAT AND PROTEIN	processed meats
	  containing wheat
	  or HFCS
			beef
			chicken
			duck
			eggs
			fish
			game meats
			lamb
			pork
			seafood
			turkey

FOODS TO ENJOY AND AVOID ▶

Food Group	Foods to Eliminate (High-FODMAP)	Foods to Enjoy in Moderation (Moderate-FODMAP)	Foods to Enjoy (1 serving per meal) (Low-FODMAP)
CONDIMENTS	condiments containing wheat or HFCS (such as barbecue sauce) ketchup mayonnaise mustard teriyaki sauce tomato paste	balsamic vinegar (1 tablespoon)	fish sauce garlic-infused oil (page 202) lemon juice lime juice oils gluten-free oyster sauce vinegar (champagne, red wine, rice wine, sherry, white wine vinegar) gluten-free soy sauce gluten-free tamari
HERBS AND SPICES	garlic powder garlic salt onion powder onion salt spice mixes containing wheat, onion, or garlic (curry powders, chili powders, etc.)	allspice (1 teaspoon) cinnamon (1 teaspoon) onion-free, garlic-free, and gluten-free chili powder (1 teaspoon) cumin (1 teaspoon)	basil bay leaves caraway cayenne chervil chile peppers chives cilantro coriander dill ginger mint mustard seeds oregano paprika parsley pepper red pepper flakes rosemary salt thyme turmeric

▸ FOODS TO ENJOY AND AVOID

Food Group	Foods to Eliminate (High-FODMAP)	Foods to Enjoy in Moderation (Moderate-FODMAP)	Foods to Enjoy (1 serving per meal) (Low-FODMAP)
SWEETENERS	agave agave nectar HFCS honey isomalt mannitol sorbitol xylitol	pure maple syrup (2 tablespoons)	acesulfame-potassium (acesulfame-k) aspartame brown sugar sucrose granulated sugar powdered sugar

Appendix B
10 Tips for Eating Out

Dining in restaurants can be stressful when you are on any kind of restricted diet, but the low-FODMAP diet can be especially difficult to adapt for eating out, since FODMAPs are found in so many common, everyday foods. But rest assured, there are many ways in which you can adapt your restaurant-dining experience that will keep your symptoms under control.

1. Plan ahead. Most restaurants nowadays post their menus online, and chain restaurants even list ingredients and nutritional information. If you are unsure of what ingredients might be in a dish, don't hesitate to call the restaurant and ask. This way you can avoid feeling as if you are boring your dining companions or subjecting your server to an inquisition when it's time to place your order.

2. Tell the waiter about your dietary restrictions. Servers and chefs are often more than happy to work with customers to accommodate their dietary restrictions, so be clear with your waiter about what you can and cannot eat, and ask for recommendations.

3. Ask questions about the menu and don't be afraid to ask more questions. If the server doesn't know what's in a dish, he or she should check with the chef.

4. Choose off-peak hours. Servers and cooks are likely to be most accommodating about answering questions or working with dietary restrictions when they aren't slammed with other customers.

5. Order simple menu items. For example, you're less likely to encounter FODMAPs if you order a steak, steamed vegetables, and a baked potato than if you order a more complicated dish like soup, stew, risotto, or a dish with a complex sauce.

6. Don't assume a dish is safe. Even if you've ordered something simple, like a steak and baked potato, check to make sure that it won't be cooked with common seasonings like onions or garlic. Ask before ordering and again when it is delivered to the table.

7. If you don't get what you asked for, don't be shy about sending it back. Be polite, but stand your ground in order to assert your dietary needs.

8. If you order a salad, ask for oil and vinegar on the side instead of dressing. Salad dressings almost always contain high-FODMAP ingredients, so don't risk it. Olive oil and red wine or white wine vinegar are FODMAP free.

9. Use a low-FODMAP smartphone app to check unfamiliar ingredients. The Monash University Low-FODMAP Diet app is frequently updated as researchers continue to test foods for FODMAPs.

10. Order items à la carte. If no composed dishes on the menu conform to your dietary needs, order a few sides, a salad, or appetizers that will. By ordering à la carte, you can create a balanced meal that won't compromise your dietary restrictions.

Appendix C
Conversion Tables

Volume Equivalents (Liquid)

US STANDARD	US STANDARD (OUNCES)	METRIC (APPROXIMATE)
2 tablespoons	1 fl. oz.	30 mL
¼ cup	2 fl. oz.	60 mL
½ cup	4 fl. oz.	120 mL
1 cup	8 fl. oz.	240 mL
1½ cups	12 fl. oz.	355 mL
2 cups or 1 pint	16 fl. oz.	475 mL
4 cups or 1 quart	32 fl. oz.	1 L
1 gallon	128 fl. oz.	4 L

Oven Temperatures

FAHRENHEIT (F)	CELSIUS (C) (APPROXIMATE)
250°	120°
300°	150°
325°	165°
350°	180°
375°	190°
400°	200°
425°	220°
450°	230°

Volume Equivalents (Dry)

US STANDARD	METRIC (APPROXIMATE)
⅛ teaspoon	.5 mL
¼ teaspoon	1 mL
½ teaspoon	2 mL
¾ teaspoon	4 mL
1 teaspoon	5 mL
1 tablespoon	15 mL
¼ cup	59 mL
⅓ cup	79 mL
½ cup	118 mL
⅔ cup	156 mL
¾ cup	177 mL
1 cup	235 mL
2 cups or 1 pint	475 mL
3 cups	700 mL
4 cups or 1 quart	1 L
½ gallon	2 L
1 gallon	4 L

Weight Equivalents

US STANDARD	METRIC (APPROXIMATE)
½ ounce	15 g
1 ounce	30 g
2 ounces	60 g
4 ounces	115 g
8 ounces	225 g
12 ounces	340 g
16 ounces or 1 pound	455 g

Appendix D
The Dirty Dozen and the Clean Fifteen

THE DIRTY DOZEN

Apples
Celery
Cherry tomatoes
Cucumbers
Grapes
Nectarines
Peaches
Potatoes
Snap peas (imported)
Spinach
Strawberries
Sweet bell peppers

The following do not meet traditional "Dirty Dozen" ranking criteria but they frequently test positive for particularly toxic pesticides:

Kale/collard greens
Hot peppers

THE CLEAN FIFTEEN

Asparagus
Avocados
Cabbage
Cantaloupes
Cauliflower
Eggplants
Grapefruits
Kiwis
Mangoes
Onions
Papayas
Pineapples
Sweet corn
Sweet peas (frozen)
Sweet potatoes

Each year the Environmental Working Group (EWG), an environmental watchdog organization based in the United States, publishes two lists of produce that they call "The Dirty Dozen" and "The Clean Fifteen." Use these lists to help minimize your exposure to chemical pesticides and fertilizers, but don't be deterred from eating conventionally grown produce on the Dirty Dozen list. The health benefits of a diet rich in fruits and vegetables outweigh the risks of pesticide exposure.

"The Dirty Dozen" are fruits and vegetables that, when conventionally grown, carry the highest residues of chemical pesticides and fertilizers. If you need to prioritize which organic produce to buy, then start with the fruits and vegetables on this list.

"The Clean Fifteen" are fruits and vegetables that, when conventionally grown, still contain very low levels of chemical pesticide or fertilizer residue. This does not mean they are pesticide-free, though, so wash these fruits and vegetables thoroughly.

Resources

The following books, websites, and apps will help you maintain a low-FODMAP diet and keep up with the latest research and developments in the field.

Books

Angelone, Anne. *The FODMAP-Free Paleo Breakthrough: 4 Weeks of Auto-immune Paleo Recipes without FODMAPs*. Seattle, WA: CreateSpace, 2013.

Bolen, Barbara, and Kathleen Bradley. *The Everything Guide To The Low-FODMAP Diet: A Healthy Plan for Managing IBS and Other Digestive Disorders*. Avon, MA: Adams Media, 2014.

Catsos, Patsy. *Flavor without FODMAPs Cookbook: Love the Foods That Love You Back*. Portland, ME: Pond Cove Press, 2014.

Catsos, Patsy. *IBS: Free at Last! Change Your Carbs, Change Your Life with the FODMAP Elimination Diet*. 2nd ed. Portland, ME: Pond Cove Press, 2012.

The FODMAP Solution: A Low FODMAP Diet Plan and Cookbook to Manage IBS and Improve Digestion. Berkeley, CA: Shasta Press, 2014.

Low-FODMAP 28-Day Plan: A Healthy Cookbook with Gut-Friendly Recipes for IBS Relief. Berkeley, CA: Rockridge Press, 2014.

Nott, Natalie, and Geoff Nott. *The Low-FODMAP Cookbook*. Mitcham, Australia: Natalie Nott, 2013.

Perazzini, Suzanne. *Low-FODMAP Menus for Irritable Bowel Syndrome: Menus for Those on a Low-FODMAP Diet*. Seattle, WA: CreateSpace, 2014.

Scarlata, Kate. *The Complete Idiot's Guide to Eating Well with IBS*. New York: Alpha Books, 2010.

Shepherd, Sue. *The Low-FODMAP Diet Cookbook: 150 Simple, Flavorful, Gut-Friendly Recipes to Ease the Symptoms of IBS, Celiac Disease, Crohn's Disease, Ulcerative Colitis, and Other Digestive Disorders.* New York: The Experiment, 2014.

Shepherd, Sue, and Peter Gibson. *The Complete Low-FODMAP Diet: A Revolutionary Plan for Managing IBS and Other Digestive Disorders.* New York: The Experiment, 2013.

Websites

Monash University. "Low-FODMAP Diet for Irritable Bowel Syndrome." www.med.monash.edu/cecs/gastro/fodmap.

"IBS Diets: FODMAP Diet Guide." www.ibsdiets.org/fodmap-diet/fodmap-food-list.

"Living FODMAP-Free for Gastrointestinal Health: Stanford University—Low-FODMAP Diet." fodmapliving.com/the-science/stanford-university-low-fodmap-diet.

Scarlata, Kate. "Kate Scarlata, RDN." Offers IBS, FODMAP diet, celiac, and diabetes counseling. www.katescarlata.com.

Shepherd, Sue. "Shepherd Works: Low-FODMAP Diet." shepherdworks.com.au/disease-information/low-fodmap-diet.

Apps

Monash University. "Low FODMAP Smartphone App." http://www.med.monash.edu/cecs/gastro/fodmap/iphone-app.html.

Mark Patrick Media. FODMAP Diet: 200 Easy Recipes. itunes.apple.com/us/app/fodmap-diet/id733235698?mt=8.

References

Celiac Disease Foundation. "What Is Celiac Disease?" Accessed November 7, 2014. celiac.org/celiac-disease/what-is-celiac-disease.

Crohn's and Colitis Foundation of America. "Diet and Nutrition." February 6, 2014. Accessed November 7, 2014. www.ccfa.org/resources/diet-and-nutrition.html.

International Foundation for Functional Gastrointestinal Disorders (IFFGD). "IBS Diet." Accessed November 7, 2014. www.aboutibs.org/site/treatment/diet.

Mayo Clinic. "Diseases and Conditions: Irritable Bowel Syndrome." July 31, 2014. Accessed November 7, 2014. www.mayoclinic.org/diseases-conditions/irritable-bowel-syndrome/basics/definition/con-20024578.

Mayo Clinic. "Diseases and Conditions: Irritable Bowel Disease." September 27, 2014. Accessed February 7, 2015. http://www.mayoclinic.org/diseases-conditions/inflammatory-bowel-disease/basics/definition/con-20034908.

Monash University Medicine, Nursing, and Health Sciences. "Low-FODMAP Diet for Irritable Bowel Syndrome." Accessed December 19, 2014. www.med.monash.edu/cecs/gastro/fodmap.

National Institute of Diabetes and Digestive and Kidney Diseases. "Celiac Disease." Accessed January 22, 2015. http://www.niddk.nih.gov/health-information/health-topics/digestive-diseases/celiac-disease/Pages/facts.aspx#other.

University of California San Francisco Medical Center. "Nutrition Tips for Inflammatory Bowel Disease." Accessed November 7, 2014. www.ucsfhealth.org/education/nutrition_tips_for_inflammatory_bowel_disease.

Weston A. Price Foundation. "Why Broth is Beautiful: Essential Roles for Proline, Glycine and Gelatin." June 18, 2003. Accessed February 2, 2015. www.westonaprice.org/health-topics/why-broth-is-beautiful-essential-roles-for-proline-glycine-and-gelatin.

Recipe Index

Index